EXERCISES FOR
HEALTHY JOINTS

D0033483

William Smith

With Contributions by Jo Brielyn
Foreword by Mary Jane Myslinski, PT, EdD

》 hatherleigh

Exercises for Healthy Joints

Hatherleigh Press is committed to preserving and protecting the natural resources of the Earth. Environmentally responsible and sustainable practices are embraced within the company's mission statement. Hatherleigh Press is a member of the Publishers Earth Alliance, committed to preserving and protecting the natural resources of the planet while developing a sustainable business model for the book publishing industry.

This book was edited and designed in the village of Hobart, New York. Hobart is a community that has embraced books and publishing as a component of its livelihood. There are several unique bookstores in the village. For more information, please visit www.hobartbookvillage.com.

www.hatherleighpress.com

Library of Congress Cataloging-in-Publication Data is available.
ISBN: 978-1-57826-344-8

All Hatherleigh Press titles are available for bulk purchase, special promotions, and premiums. For information about reselling and special purchase opportunities, please call 1-800-528-2550 and ask for the Special Sales Manager.

Cover Design by Heather Daugherty
Interior Design by Nick Macagnone
Photography by Catarina Astrom

10 9 8 7 6 5 4 3 2 1

Printed in the United States

Disclaimer
Consult your physician before beginning any exercise program. The author and publisher of this book and workout disclaim any liability, personal or professional, resulting from the misapplication of any of the following procedures described in this publication.

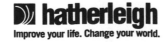

Table of Contents

FOREWORD

Unfortunately, as we grow older our strength often decreases, leading to joint pain. As a physical therapist, I know the importance of maintaining good joint and muscle health. *Exercises for Healthy Joints* explains, in everyday language, how to do this by following clearly delineated programs that can work for you.

William Smith has done an excellent job in taking basic scientific explanations of the joints and their structures, and paring them down so that everyone can learn these concepts. It is important to have an understanding of joint anatomy so that the exercises can be done correctly and in a safe manner. As is clearly stated throughout this book, pain is not the end goal!

Throughout the book, Smith provides an overview of current evidence-based medicine to explain why the techniques and procedures in this book are effective in improving joint health. *Exercises for Healthy Joints* also includes information on the latest research to demonstrate the many benefits of exercise and how it can help in modifying chronic diseases.

The programs described in the following pages have been designed for anyone with joint pain (or anyone who aims to prevent the development of joint pain). The exercises are easy to follow and will be very beneficial for all that keep up with the programs. Because each exercise has been specially selected for joint health, they are sure to help improve movement and build muscle strength, which can ultimately enhance overall quality of life for those suffering from joint pain.

When exercising, always keep in mind the safety points that are provided in this book—safety is your number one priority. If any exercise or movement is causing you pain, please consult your physician or physical therapist. The physical therapist can treat the pain and modify the program so that you can continue down the path of continued health.

—*Mary Jane Myslinski, PT, MA, Ed.D.*

CHAPTER ONE

About the Knees, Shoulders, Hips, and Ankles

The joints are the crossroads of movement. Without our joints, we wouldn't be able to sit, walk, or run. Joints everywhere in our body allow us to perform a wide variety of complex movements from walking to the store to running a marathon. Although many of us may not be aware, guarding the health of our joints is vital to daily functioning and physical fitness. As we age, this becomes even more important.

There are many different types of joints throughout the body, ranging from the small joints that make up the knuckles in your hands to the large joints in the lower body. There is even a joint in your neck that allows your head to move from side to side. This book focuses on the joints which most often cause pain in the human body: the knees, shoulders, hips, and ankles. As we age, these joints in particular can become damaged or injured if not treated properly. Now, with most people living longer than ever, an increase in life expectancy means more individuals may experience pain. According to the Centers for Disease Control, by 2030, nearly one-fifth of Americans will be in their sixties or older. Taking steps to protect these joints well into the senior years is becoming more and more important.

How Joints Function

A *joint* is defined as the area where two or more bones make contact. Joints provide structural support of the mass of the body as well as enabling movement.

Joints are classified based on both structure and function. Structural classification refers to how the bones connect. Functional classification pertains to what the joint does in the body; in other words, what type of movement the joint enables.

There are three ways to classify joints by structure, based on the bones:
- **Fibrous Joints:** This type of joint connects bones together, but does not allow for movement. The skull and pelvis both consist of areas of bones that are held together by fibrous joints. A fibrous joint consists of dense, collagen-rich tissue.
- **Cartilaginous Joints:** These joints allow for a small range of movement. In a cartilaginous joint, bones are held together by cartilage. The spine and ribs are both cartilaginous joints.
- **Synovial Joints:** These joints allow for a great range of movement because the bones are not directly joined. Empty areas between the bones, called *synovial cavities*, are filled with synovial fluid, which helps to lubricate and prevent the bones from rubbing against each other. The hips and the knees are both synovial joints.

The functional classifications, which describe the type of movement a joint allows, are:
- **Synarthrosis:** This type of joint permits little or no movement. Most synarthrosis joints are fibrous joints.
- **Amphiarthrosis:** This joint allows for some mobility. Cartilaginous joints are categorized as amphiarthosis.
- **Diarthrosis:** This type of joint allows a great degree of movement. All diarthrosis joints are synovial. This includes the hips, shoulders, elbows, and knees.

Common Terms Related to Movement of Joints

A more specific description of the type of movement enabled by a joint can also be helpful. This book uses many of the terms below to describe the body's joints as it relates to how they enable the body to move.

- **Pivot Joints:** A pivot joint allows for rotation around an axis. The neck is a pivot joint that allows the head to turn.
- **Ball and Socket Joints:** A ball and socket joint, where the rounded area of one bone "fits" into a depression of the other, makes radial movement possible. The hips and shoulders are both ball and socket joints.
- **Ellipsoid Joints:** These joints allow the same type of movement as a ball and socket joint, only with a more limited range of movement. The wrist is an ellipsoid joint.
- **Saddle Joints:** A saddle joint does not make rotation possible, but instead allows for movement back and forth and up and down.
- **Hinge Joints:** A hinge joint makes extension and retraction of a limb possible.

Anatomy of the Joints

Although the joint is defined as the area where bones meet, movement would not be possible without connective tissues and fluids to cushion and control the bones. Stability of a joint is provided by *ligaments* which prevent the joint from dislocating. Ligaments serve as bridges between one bone and another.

Cartilage is fibrous elastic tissue that cushions the area between the joints and prevents bones from rubbing or grinding together. Cartilage also absorbs shock. Without cartilage, we would not be able to bend and twist.

Cartilage thins and wears out over the years. It is damaged easily and has a very limited ability for self-restoration. When cartilage does restore itself, as sometimes occurs after an injury, the cartilage that replaces the old is usually more prone to tearing and cracking.

The Knee

The knee joins the thigh with the leg. The knee is a very complex joint, known as a *mobile trocho-ginglymus*; in other words, a pivotal hinge joint. The knee is classified as a synovial joint and has cavities that are filled with synovial fluid to cushion the bones. The knee is the largest joint in the human body and supports almost the entire weight of the body. It also allows for flexion, extension, and slight rotation.

There are two types of cartilage in the knee: fibrous cartilage (also called meniscus) and hyaline cartilage. Fibrous cartilage resists pressure, whereas hyaline cartilage covers the surface where the joints interact to allow for smooth movement. At birth, a baby has cartilage over the knee area in place of the bone of the kneecap. The kneecap is later formed by the age of three in females and by the age of five in males.

The knee has several ligaments. Two types of ligaments in particular are crucial to the knee's functioning: the ACL (anterior cruciate ligament) and the PCL (posterior cruciate ligament). These stabilize the knee and prevent the kneecap from dislocating. In active individuals, the ACL is often torn during twisting or bending of the knee, making this a very common sports injury.

Because the knee carries so much weight, it is highly susceptible to injury and osteoarthritis. These conditions are exacerbated by weight gain. Every extra pound gained puts four times the amount of stress on the knees.

The Hips

The hip joint, scientifically referred to as the *acetabulofemoral joint,* is the joint between the femur and the pelvis. The rounded head of the femur sits in the round depression of the acetabulum of the pelvis. The hip joint is a synovial joint and helps support the weight of the body, whether the body is static or mobile. The bones of the hip area are largely covered by muscle, which means that, unlike other joints, the movements of the bones of the hip joint are not visible from outside the body.

The joint surfaces of the hip are covered in a lubricated layer called *articular hyaline cartilage*. Additionally, the hip joint is supported by five ligaments, which strengthen the joint and prevent excessive movement. The y-shaped iliofemoral ligament is the strongest in the human body.

The hips of the human body are different in males and females. In a human female, the hips are wider (the widening occurs during puberty), and the femur is spaced further apart than in males, so as to widen the opening in the hip bone and allow for childbirth.

The Ankles

The ankle joint, known as a *talocrural joint*, is formed where the foot and leg meet. The ankle connects the ends of the tibia and the fibula in the lower limb of the leg with the uppermost part of the talus bone in the foot. The ankle is a synovial hinge joint and allows for a wide range of movement in the foot.

The ankle is supported by several ligaments. The *deltoid ligament,* along with three lateral ligaments (including the *anterior talofibular ligament*), supports the joint. It is the anterior talofibular ligament which is most often involved in a sprained ankle injury. The most common ankle injuries are ankle sprains or fractures.

The Shoulders

The shoulder is made up of three bones, but the major joint of the shoulder is the *glenohumeral joint.* The shoulder consists of the clavicle (collarbone); scapula (shoulder blade) and humerus (upper arm bone), as well as muscles, ligaments and tendons. The glenohumeral joint is located where the humerus attaches to the scapula and is classified as a ball and socket joint —the "ball" is at the top of the arm bone and the "socket" is a portion of the scapula. The function of this joint is to allow for mobility. Because of the glenohumeral joint, we are able to rotate the arm in circles or move it up and away from the body.

Two kinds of cartilage aid in the functioning of the shoulder by connecting one bone to the other. White cartilage on the ends of the bones, called *articular cartilage,* allows bones to move over each other without rubbing. *Labrum cartilage,* which is stiffer, is found only around the sockets. Two sacs of fluid, called bursae, permit bones, muscles and tendons to move over each other smoothly.

The tremendous range of movement that the shoulder allows also means that it is very likely to be injured. Most injuries of the shoulder are "rotator cuff" injuries, which occur around the group of muscles and the tendons that act to stabilize the shoulder.

What is Joint Pain?

At some point, everyone has experienced joint pain. Individuals experiencing joint pain often describe it in a variety of ways. Most often, it is experienced as tenderness or discomfort due to the swelling or inflammation near the joint. Often, joint pain will lead an individual to avoid utilizing a certain area of their body, hindering movement.

Sometimes joint pain is fleeting and can be remedied without the help of a doctor. In other cases, joint pain is recurring. One of the most common conditions is arthritis and chronic joint pain. According to the Centers for Disease Control and Prevention, one in three adults in the United States suffers from arthritis or chronic joint pain.

Any person with unusual, chronic joint pain should consult a doctor. Joint pain can be diagnosed with a physical exam, patient history, and, if necessary, x-rays, bone scans, or MRI's.

In some cases, joint pain is one of many symptoms of a more serious illness, including:
- Rheumatic fever
- Mumps
- Chicken pox
- Hepatitis
- Bursitis
- Influenza
- Lupus or SLE (Systemic Lupus Erythematosus)
- Gout (if the pain occurs mostly around the feet, ankles, or legs)

Arthritis

When the cartilage that cushions and protects the joints is depleted, arthritis can develop. Without joint cartilage, bone will rub against bone, causing pain. Arthritis is defined as a condition where damaged, inflamed joints in the body cause pain, swelling, and stiffness, and may also hinder movement. In the United States, approximately 37 million people have a form of arthritis, making it the most common cause of disability.

There are over 100 types of arthritis. The most common type of arthritis is called *osteoarthritis,* also known as degenerative joint disease. Other types of arthritis include rheumatoid arthritis and psoriatic arthritis, both of which are autoimmune diseases (conditions where the body attacks itself), as well as septic arthritis, which is caused by a joint infection.

The pain caused by arthritis can be severe, and leads to hospitalization for roughly 1 million people each year. There is no cure for arthritis. Physical therapy and medication can help to assuage symptoms and manage the pain. During physical therapy, patients work to strengthen muscles to relieve some of the workload on the joints. Patients also improve flexibility to reduce the incidence of injury and learn how to minimize further damage to the joints during everyday activities. Drugs can help to reduce inflammation as well as ease pain. In some cases, surgery is necessary to repair the damaged joint.

Osteoarthritis

Osteoarthritis occurs after trauma or injury to the joint, infection, or simply due to the aging process. It is also known as "wear and tear" arthritis because repetitive activity can cause joint cartilage to break down and lead to this condition. The larger joints of the body, including the hips, back, or knees, are most affected by osteoarthritis. The cause of osteoarthritis is not well understood, but injury, age, and genetics are believed to be contributing factors. Because osteoarthritis is the result of wear to the body and depends in large part on someone's lifestyle and treatment of their body, osteoarthritis can afflict individuals at any age, although it is most likely to manifest itself after the age of 40.

Facts about Osteoarthritis

- About 21 million adults have osteoarthritis
- The condition can affect anyone
- Osteoarthritis occurs more often as we age
- For women, osteoarthritis is more common after age 50
- For men, the incidence of osteoarthritis often occurs before age 45
- Almost twice as many women as men suffer from arthritis
- The area of most pain due to osteoarthritis varies; for women, the hands, knees, ankles, and feet are most affected; for men, pain typically occurs in the wrists, hips, and spine
- Arthritis accounts for nearly forty million doctor visits and more than half a million hospitalizations
- 285,000 children under age seventeen have arthritis, including 50,000 who have juvenile rheumatoid arthritis

Osteoporosis

Osteoporosis is a bone disease that causes low bone mass and deterioration or weakening of the bone, making fractures more likely. Osteoporosis is classified as either primary or secondary: *primary osteoporosis* is bone loss due to aging, whereas *secondary osteoporosis* is caused by outside factors, such as certain side effects of specific medications, poor nutrition, or chronic medical conditions. Osteoporosis is the most common bone disease and it affects both men and women. In the United States, close to 30 million people are affected by osteoporosis. About 1.5 million of these individuals experience bone fracture, including vertebral fractures, hip fractures, and wrist fractures. Currently, the elderly are most affected by osteoporosis. As the lifespan of the average American continues to increase, it is estimated that osteoporosis diagnoses will continue to rise.

Osteoporosis can go unrecognized for years, usually only making itself known once someone experiences a fall or fracture. This is most often when an osteoporosis diagnosis is made. However, a test that measures *bone mineral density (BMD)* can also be used to assess whether or not someone has osteoporosis. Doctors often recommend measuring BMD in women over the age of 65, as well as those with risk factors, including family history, a history of broken bones, and smoking.

As stated, cartilage has limited capacity for renewal and regeneration. Cartilage can be further damaged by inflammation. During an injury, the area of the body that is damaged most often becomes inflamed. Inflammation disrupts the structure of the joints on a biomechanical level. In other words, the inflammatory cells involved in inflammation release chemicals destructive to cartilage.

The Importance of Exercise

Exercise is key to maintaining healthy joints. This is because, as we age, muscle mass decreases. If we don't exercise to maintain muscle mass, the joint (instead of the muscle) will end up doing most of the work. The joint will absorb impact, pounding, and shock, gradually becoming damaged.

In addition to building important muscle mass, exercise also reduces stiffness in the joints, strengthens bones, reduces pain, and improves flexibility and balance. Exercise also keeps tendons and ligaments elastic. The exercises in this book encourage a wide variety of low-impact movement to avoid overuse of the joints and encourage flexibility and improved muscle mass.

Exercise is also important to keep body weight in check. When we gain excess weight, the joints of the body have to carry a heavier load and do more work. This means the joint will undergo damage over the long term. As mentioned, the knees in particular will experience more damage over time for those individuals who do not maintain a healthy weight.

It can be encouraging to know that even a small amount of weight loss can make a big difference. For example, losing as little as 11 pounds may improve joint health of the knee and reduce the risk of osteoarthritis of the knee by 50 percent. For women, losing a little over ten pounds can cut arthritis pain in half.

Exercise and Joint Pain

How should people who are experiencing pain, either due to arthritis or injury, approach physical fitness? First, seek the advice of a doctor. Communicate to him or her which exercise or movements cause you the most pain. Then, you can develop a physical fitness regimen with these restrictions in mind. A doctor may recommend that you allow your body to rest or at least reduce the intensity and frequency of your workout.

Be aware that if you are experiencing pain in a specific joint, exercise can still be beneficial if you take the right approach. For those with minor pain, exercising the joint can actually be helpful to the body. Exercise helps to deliver nutrients to various areas in the body, while also flushing out debris and toxins. Exercise also reduces stress levels. Stress produces a hormone called *cortisol* in the body, which further exacerbates inflammation (which can damage cartilage), so any reduction in stress is helpful.

Low-impact ways to exercise and build muscle include:
- **Weight Training:** Light weights or isometric exercise reduces impact and stress on the joints, while also building muscle.
- **Stretching:** Stretching relaxes the tendons that surround the joint and improve mobility. Yoga, pilates, and tai chi are all excellent stretching

exercises.

- **Endurance Exercises:** Biking, walking, swimming, and tennis encourage the joints to work and reduces the likelihood of injury.

We will take a closer look at specific exercises and healthy living guidelines in Chapters 3 and 6.

CHAPTER TWO

What the New Studies Say

Recent research makes it abundantly clear that exercise is the key to guarding the health of your joints. Not only does exercise keep your body weight down, as mentioned in the last chapter, but it is vital for keeping your joints strong and your cartilage and ligaments flexible and healthy. This is true for men and women of all ages. It has been shown that even those with joint pain or arthritis have a lower incidence of symptoms and improved quality of life when they exercise regularly.

Exercise for older individuals can help prevent problems later on in life. In Australia, a study examined the effects of exercise for middle-aged women as well as senior citizens over a three-year period. The study found that women in their 70's who exercised for 75 minutes each week reduced the odds of developing arthritis symptoms. The results were even better when the women exercised more; those who participated in moderate physical activity for 150 minutes each week reduced the chances of arthritis even further.

Exercise is particularly helpful for those with arthritis. As published in the *Journal of Rehabilitation Medicine* in 2009, researchers in Sweden found that individuals with rheumatoid arthritis who exercised their hands over a six-week period improved hand strength and dexterity. Staying physically fit is recommended for those with chronic arthritis. The publication *Current Opinion in Rheumatology* reported in 2009 that "there is a preponderance of strong scientific evidence that both aerobic and muscle strengthening exercises, alone or in combination, are safe and moderately effective for individuals with chronic arthritis." Among the benefits reported were improved fitness, mobility, and function, as well as a reduction in symptoms.

One of the reasons why exercise is so helpful for those with arthritis is that effective exercise does not have to be high-impact. A 2007 study conducted by Flavia M. Cicuttini, Ph.D., of Monash University and Alfred Hospital in Australia concluded that even low-impact activity (such as walking) is sufficient to prevent osteoarthritis by strengthening cartilage and improving bone mass. They concluded, "Our data suggest that at least 20 minutes once per week of activity sufficient to result in sweating or some shortness of breath might be adequate."

Consistency is essential to getting the most benefit from exercise. Researchers from the Department of Immunology/Rheumatology at Stanford University, along with scientists from Genentech biomedical company, examined the effect of exercise in men and women over 50 years of age, over a fourteen-year period. They determined that regularity and routine is key. In the study, regular exercise reduced pain for patients with osteoarthritis in the knees and also prevented lower back pain. It should also be noted that patients who did not participate in regular physical activity experienced negative results. Not only were they more prone to injury, but they showed lower bone density and weakened muscle tone. The researchers concluded,

> The primary finding from this investigation is that while pain does increase with age in subjects in all study groups, there was no progressive increase in musculoskeletal pain in older adults who participated in regular vigorous exercise, including running, compared with those who did not. Initial differences favoring exercisers were shown to be maintained over time. As pain and disability are linked, our findings add to the evidence that morbidity associated with aging can be reduced by participating in regular aerobic activity.

Treatment Options: Surgery

If all other forms of treatment fail to address joint pain, surgery may be necessary. Each year, more than 770,000 hip and knee replacements are performed in the United States. Although surgeries are common, a doctor should work carefully with a patient to determine if surgery is the only option. Physical exams and thorough diagnostic testing, as well as further tests to closely examine the bones, include:

- A radiograph or x-ray, which is useful for revealing fractures or other damage to the bone.
- A computed tomography, or CAT scan, which generates three-dimensional images of the joints.
- Magnetic resonance imaging (MRI), which uses a large magnet, radio waves, and a computer to generate a picture of the joint. MRI's can reveal ligament injuries, as well as damage to the tendons and bones.

Kinesiology and Orthopedics

Kinesiology, or human kinetics, is the science of human movement. Kinesiology is most often applied in rehabilitation professions, such as physical and occupational therapy. Kinesiology is also applied in sports medicine and in the exercise industry. The sciences of biomechanics, anatomy, physiology, psychology, and neuroscience all play a role in kinesiology. It should be noted that although the term *kinesiologist* is not a professional designation or license to practice, the study of kinesiology is often a basis for obtaining degrees in the fields of physiology or neuroscience.

Orthopedics is a field of medicine that addresses disorders of the musculoskeletal system. Orthopedic doctors treat conditions such as osteoporosis and arthritis, as well as trauma to the bones, including injury, degenerative diseases, infections, or tumors. Treatment can involve both surgical and non-surgical means.

Ankle Surgery

It is estimated that, in 2010, about 4,400 surgeries will be performed to replace arthritic or injured ankles with artificial joints. The two most common types of surgery involving the ankle are ankle fusion, also known as *ankle arthrodesis,* and ankle replacement. Either surgery may be performed after all other options have been exhausted. Individuals who often have ankle surgery are those would have arthritis or a worn-out and painful ankle caused by serious injury or fracture.

In an ankle fusion surgery, cartilage is removed from both sides of the joint so that bone will fuse onto bone. The ankle is kept in place during healing using a metal frame placed outside the body. It usually takes about 12-15 weeks for the bones to fuse. In ankle replacement surgery, the ankle joint surface is replaced with an artificial implant. A bone graft is often used to encourage the bones to fuse.

Today, many doctors practice a procedure called *arthroscopy* to help diagnose joint problems, repair joints during surgery, and monitor healing after surgery. In an arthroscopy, the surgeon is able to view joints and the surrounding soft tissues by inserting a small viewing instrument into the area near the affected joint. Arthroscopy is a very common procedure when examining or operating on the knees, shoulders, and ankles.

Hip Replacement Surgery

According to the American Academy of Orthopedic Surgeons, more than 231,000 total hip replacements are performed each year in the United States. About 85% of artificial hip joints last 20 years before the components begin to break down and the joint needs to be replaced. In a hip replacement surgery, an artificial hip joint is implanted. Currently, there are two ways to perform hip replacement surgery: either traditionally, or using a minimally invasive procedure.

During standard hip replacement surgery, the "ball" and "socket" of the joint is removed and replaced with new, artificial joints. After surgery, the patient stays in the hospital for four to six days, where weeks-long physical therapy begins. It should be noted that the replacement hip joint is meant only to aid with day-to-day movement; those with artificial hips should avoid sports or heavy activity.

Knee Surgery

According to the American Academy of Orthopedic Surgeons, over 250,000 knee replacement surgeries, or *arthroplasties,* are performed in the United States each year. Most of these surgeries are for individuals over the age of 65. However, more and more surgeries are being performed on younger patients. The first knee replacement was performed in 1968. Since then, advances in surgical technique as well as replacement knees have changed the field of knee replacement surgeries.

The complexity of knee replacement surgery depends on whether one knee or both knees are being replaced. In cases of those afflicted with arthritis (who usually have pain in both knees) both knees are often replaced at one time, rather than having two separate surgeries. In other cases, doctors recommend operating on one knee at a time so that the unaffected leg can aid movement while the leg that was operated on heals itself. Replacing both knees is known as *bilateral total knee replacement,* or *bilateral knee arthroplasty.*

During knee surgery, the damaged part of the joint is removed and the surface of the bone is replaced so that an artificial joint can be attached. A period of four to five months of physical therapy is required after knee surgery, a process which begins when the patient is still in the hospital after surgery. Individuals who have had surgery can engage in low-impact physical activity, such as swimming or walking, and can eventually select high-impact sports.

Shoulder Surgery

In the United States, approximately 7,000 total shoulder replacements were performed each year from 1996 through 2002. Generally, shoulder damage can be treated without surgery. However, if the pain continues to be severe and the shoulder does not respond to treatment over a period of three to six months, surgery may be advised. One of the most common surgeries is to the rotator cuff. As stated earlier, this area refers to the muscles and tendons that cover the shoulder joint and hold the ball and socket joint in place. Usually, problems with the rotator cuff are the result of torn tendons, which can occur from overuse or injury.

Other specific conditions that sometimes require shoulder surgery are damage to the joint lining, usually as a result of arthritis, as well as torn ligaments or a loose shoulder joint. A surgeon will take a close look at the cartilage, bones, tendons and ligaments of the shoulder to assess damage before repairing damaged tissues.

In shoulder surgery, damaged tissue around the rotator cuff is replaced. Recovery time after surgery varies, usually from one to six months, during which time physical therapy is important to ensure the full range of movement is regained. Individuals who have had shoulder surgery can return to physical activity and playing sports after a period of time.

CHAPTER THREE

Long-Term Joint Health

Not long ago, it was assumed that losing muscle, mass, bone, and flexibility was a natural part of the aging process. However, more recent research has shown that the way we choose to live our lives and treat our bodies makes all the difference when it comes to enjoying a pain-free, healthy lifestyle well into our senior years. Adopting a lifestyle with joint health in mind is more important than ever.

The first step is to watch your waistline. Adopt good eating and exercise habits. When deciding on an exercise program, consider a wide variety of options. No matter what, keep moving! Yoga, tai chi, strength training,

For those with joint pain, consider alternative practices such as yoga or qi gong. Both practices use focused breathing and slow, controlled movements in helping to reduce stress and improve flexibility and muscle tone.

Pilates, water exercises, tennis, elliptical training, cycling, golf, and dancing are all good choices. Walking as little as 30 minutes—even ten minutes three times a day—can alleviate joint pain, improve mobility, and reduce fatigue.

If you become injured during exercise, icing the damaged joint can help in the short-term. When you exercise, synovial fluid lubricates the joints, which aids movement. However, if this fluid remains near the joint for too long after activity, it can crack cartilage. Ice helps encourage the synovial fluid to flush out away from the joint and into the lymphatic system. Try using ice for ten minutes on sore joints after exercise.

Everyday Tips for Joint Health

Wear sensible shoes and avoid high heels. A three-inch heel causes seven times more stress to the foot than a one-inch heel. High heels also put more stress on the knees. Instead, choose comfortable shoes with little or no heel.

If you have a job that requires you to sit for most of the day, be sure to take a break every 30 minutes to stand up. It is harmful to the body to be in one position for a long period of time.

If you have to handle something heavy, use the muscles in your legs to lift the weight, rather than lifting with your back. Holding items close to your body is also less stressful for the joints. If possible, slide objects instead of lifting them.

When working at a computer, take advantage of document holders. These help to keep information at eye-level so that your neck does not become strained from looking down repeatedly. Sit 20-26 inches from the computer monitor to properly align the head, arms, hands and wrists and reduce pain.

The Importance of Eating Right

In addition to exercise, a balanced diet is essential to maintaining a healthy body weight. When it comes to joint health, a nutritional approach focuses on supporting and promoting the production of synovial fluid and cartilage, which helps to reduce inflammation.

The following foods will help to guard joint health for years to come:

- **Salmon & other oily fish (mackerel, sardines, herring, fresh tuna, trout, kippers, anchovies, halibut):** In addition to being a good source of protein and vitamin D, these foods contain a high amount of omega 3 fats, which have anti-inflammatory effects. It has been shown that these types of seafood ease symptoms of both osteoarthritis and rheumatoid arthritis.
- **Ginger:** Ginger root contains *gingerols*, active components that are thought to prevent the body from producing inflammatory substances. For a delicious and easy way to take in ginger's benefits, try adding fresh ginger root to hot lemon and water, or to curries, stir fries, breads and cookies.
- **Turmeric:** Turmeric contains the potent ingredient *curcumin* which is thought to protect against inflammation. Curcumin may also help to alleviate arthritis pain and stiffness. Add turmeric to curries, tagines and soups.
- **Cherries:** Cherries are rich in antioxidants that can help prevent and repair the damage caused by free radicals. Additionally, *flavonoids* present in cherries prevent inflammation and reduce levels of uric acid in painful joints.
- **Beta carotene-rich foods (sweet potato, carrots, kale, melon, mango, butternut squash, papaya, cantaloupe, apricots):** Carotenes such as *beta-cryptoxanthin* lessen inflammation and help reduce the pain of rheumatoid arthritis.
- **Nuts and seeds:** Nuts and seeds feature vitamin E, essential fats, zinc, and biotin, which are all vital nutrients valued for producing anti-inflammatory *prostaglandins.* Try a wide variety such as walnuts, pumpkin seeds, flaxseed, sunflower seeds, sesame seeds, almonds, cashews, and Brazil nuts.
- **Berries:** Berries have a high level of vitamin C, a key nutrient for the production of collagen, a major component of cartilage. Berries also feature anti-inflammatory *bioflavonoids*, which help inhibit enzymes that break down collagen. If possible, eat a cup of berries every day.
- **Oats and whole grains (brown rice, quinoa, lentils, dark green leafy vegetables):** These foods are great sources of magnesium, which is important for the production of *hyaluronic acid,* a major component in synovial fluid as well as cartilage.
- **Dairy (milk, cheese, yogurt):** These foods are rich in calcium, which is important for healthy bones. They also feature magnesium, folic acid

and vitamins, which are beneficial for a healthy system. Seek out low-fat or skim dairy products to avoid saturated fat, which can exacerbate inflammation.

The Dangers of Dehydration

Difficulty concentrating, fatigue, and stiffness in body tissues may be caused by dehydration. The general recommendation is six to eight glasses of water per day, yet with elderly populations this amount is easily decreased by one to two glasses. Low hydration is a concern even in inactive populations that do not physically exert themselves beyond activities of daily living. Basic physiological functions including digestion, perspiration, urination, and renal function all require fluids.

General Health Tips

- Whenever possible, seek out organic foods. Organic fresh fruits and vegetables are less likely to contain pesticides or other harsh chemicals.
- Consuming enough water is key to maintaining a healthy body. The human body is 60% water, and the brain is 80% water. Our entire body needs water in order to function.
- If you are smoking, be aware that smoking leads to lower bone density, an increased risk factor for osteoporosis and other bone-related conditions.
- Be sure to get enough sleep. Cellular regeneration takes place when we sleep and is vital to staying healthy.

Stress Relievers: Breathing, Meditation, and Visual Imagery

Ask yourself, "How many times has my joint pain flared up when I have been under an enormous amount of stress?" Chances are that in today's day and age every one of us has experienced stress at some point either consciously or subconsciously.

Controlling stress helps the body to fully realize the full benefit of regular physical activities. One method that has been shown to enhance mental acuity, focus, and brain function are "mind-body" connection exercises.

How Stress Happens and Why it Affects Joint Health

Stress is a normal physiological response in the human body. As such, stress that causes pain can actually be a good thing in some situations! Pain and discomfort tells your body that something is not quite right. In *Exercises for Healthy Joints* we do not want any pain during the execution of exercises, but you might notice muscle fatigue and soreness. This is normal. When you exercise, be aware of when and how your body feels physical stress. Pain is a signal to stop a particular exercise.

Emotional or psychological stress presents in many forms including work, family, and that darn traffic you sit in everyday. Stress can be good (eustress) or bad (distress). Hence, jubilation during your daughter's wedding can be a good stress, yet similar to the same response you will have during a stressful meeting at work. The point is that you will have a similar physiological response and if you currently have joint pain, that pain will more than likely manifest in that spot. The connection between stress and joint pain is very real. When we are under stress, our body releases a steroid hormone called *cortisol*. When cortisol is present, the body reacts by immediately working to detoxify it. During this process, sulfate materials play a key role; they are crucial to breaking down cortisol. However, sulfate is also vital to the maintenance of healthy cartilage. When stress is present in the body and sulfates are used to break down cortisol, the reserves of sulfate used to repair cartilage are compromised. This is yet another reason why reducing stress is key to maintaining a healthy system, one that is able to function properly and maintain healthy joints.

Deep Breathing

Practice deep breathing as a form of relaxation before bed. Slow, deep breathing is an excellent way to slow the heart rate and contemplate the day's events. Focus on breathing in through the nose and out through the mouth.

Simple Stress Reliever

Looking for a simple, healthy way to help get through the day? Try breathing exercises—a wonderfully effective way to reduce stress, maintain focus, and feel energized. Exhaling completely is one breathing exercise to try—it can promote deeper breathing and better health.

Give it a try: Simply take a deep breath, let it out effortlessly, and then squeeze out a little more. Doing this regularly will help build up the muscles between your ribs, and your exhalations will soon become deeper and longer. Start by practicing this exhalation exercise consciously, and before long it will become a healthy, unconscious habit.

Daily Tips to Stay Healthy

1. Stretch for five minutes before getting out of bed in the morning to prepare your muscles for movement.

2. Drink one large glass of water in the morning to stabilize your morning eating habits. Our bodies are approximately 60% water. By replenishing our body first thing in the morning, the regulatory systems of our body, namely heart rate and blood pressure, will stay increasingly balanced.

3. Eat 300-400 calories for breakfast. Research has shown that eating breakfast improves memory performance.

4. Healthy lunch foods can easily be made to order at local restaurants. Pick steamed and broiled foods over fried. Gastro-intestinal (GI) irritability can be exacerbated by fried and processed foods.

5. Mid-afternoon is a perfect time to have a moderate carbohydrate/moderate protein-based snack or drink. An example would be a smoothie of dark berries with whey protein blended with water. If you like texture, have homemade trail mix with nuts and raisins.

6. If eating dinner around 5:00 or 6:00, it can be on the heavier side, whereas dinners at 7:00 or later should be on the lighter side. If you know you will be having dinner later in the day, add another serving of milk instead of water to your smoothie, increasing the total caloric intake for your mid-afternoon snack. This will keep you from getting hungry as the day goes on.

7. Take a walk after dinner, but wait 20-30 minutes after eating. Stimulating blood flow through aerobically-based movements that are low impact (not

running) aids in the digestive process. Giving 30 minutes allows the food to settle.

8. Write a short to-do list before going to bed. Keep your list to three priority items if you do not work and one to two priority items if you have a full-time occupation.

9. Practice deep breathing as a form of relaxation before bed. Deep breathing is an excellent way to slow the heart rate. Focus on breathing in through the nose and out through the mouth.

CHAPTER FOUR

Path to Better Health:
The Benefits of Exercise

This book is a tool for enjoying physical fitness and improving the health of your joints while also reducing the likelihood of injury. Keep in mind that every individual is different. If your body is hurting in one area, take care not to overuse it. For example, if your knees are bothering you, you'll still burn calories and get a good workout by swimming instead of running (swimming is a more low-impact activity). When your joints are feeling better, you can then resume running or other higher-impact aerobic exercises. The exercises in this book provide a wide variety of options. Try them out and see which routines work best for you.

Exercise Categories

This book's exercise program is broken down into three primary categories:
1. **Stability**
2. **Stamina**
3. **Movement**

Stability

Stability training teaches the body to stabilize the hips, back, and shoulders. We then apply strength exercises like squats or lunges, called resistance training.

Core Stability

Core training has gotten a lot of press beginning in the mid-nineties, when greater awareness of its importance began to become common knowledge. The result of core training, core strength could more appropriately be called *core stability.*

Forward bending and backward extensions occur in what is called a sagittal plane of motion. Examples of common exercises that occur in this plane are toe touches and back extensions, both of which are dynamic movements.

Planes of the Body

Sagittal Plane (Lateral Plane)

A vertical plane running from front to back; divides the body or any of its parts into right and left sides.

Coronal Plane (Frontal Plane)

A vertical plane running from side to side; divides the body or any of its parts into anterior and posterior portions.

Transverse Plane (Axial Plane)

A horizontal plane; divides the body or any of its parts into upper and lower parts.

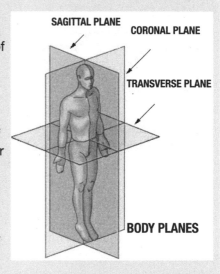

SAGITTAL PLANE   CORONAL PLANE

TRANSVERSE PLANE

BODY PLANES

Stamina

Stamina focuses on building the energy systems of the body, and involves maintaining energy and strength for a long period of time while performing a particular activity. The exercises in this book work on building one's total work capacity (functional capacity) by changing rest intervals, and incorporating circuits and functional exercises such as walking up and down stairs or picking up objects.

Developing endurance, or stamina, and work capacity are two primary goals of the exercise programs in this book. Endurance is broken down into two types, cardio-respiratory and muscular. These are defined by the Centers for Disease Control as follows:

Cardio-Respiratory Endurance

Cardio-respiratory endurance is the ability of the body's circulatory and respiratory systems to supply fuel during sustained physical activity (US-DHHS, 1996 as adapted from Corbin & Lindsey, 1994). To improve your cardio-respiratory endurance, try activities that keep your heart rate elevated at a safe level for a sustained length of time such as walking, swimming, or bicycling. The activity you choose does not have to be strenuous to improve your cardio-respiratory endurance. Start slowly with an activity you enjoy, and gradually work up to a more intense pace.

Muscular Endurance

Muscular endurance is the ability of the muscle to continue to perform without fatigue (USDHHS, 1996 as adapted from Wilmore & Costill, 1994). To improve your muscular endurance, try cardio-respiratory activities such as walking, jogging, bicycling, or dancing.

Movement

Movement consists of flexibility training, soft tissue rolling, and balance training.

The movement section of exercises focuses on increasing body temperature, improving body awareness, enhancing coordination, and self-applied soft tissue therapy. A recent *New York Times* article entitled "Stretching: The Truth" discusses the benefits of movement-based exercises for increasing overall functional capabilities. The article notes,

> A well-designed warm-up starts by increasing body heat and blood flow. Warm muscles and dilated blood vessels pull oxygen from the bloodstream more efficiently and use stored muscle fuel more effectively.

> They also withstand loads better. One significant, if gruesome, study found that the leg-muscle tissue of laboratory rabbits could be stretched farther before ripping if it had been electronically stimulated—that is, warmed up.

Foam Rolling

Myofascial treatment ("myo" meaning muscle and "fascia" meaning specialized connective tissue) can be performed throughout the body through a technique called foam rolling.

Foam rolling has shown extremely positive anecdotal results in therapy and mainstream clients, particularly those with joint pain. Remember that joint pain can be caused by a number of factors including:
* Injuries that lead to chronic pain such as osteoarthritis
* Overuse (as seen in runner's knee or tennis elbow)
* Lack of use that leads to joint stiffness

By applying the foam roller in designated areas of your body, you can alleviate the daily pain you are experiencing. Here are some areas where you can apply the foam roller:
* Upper/middle back
* Hips/glutes
* Outside of the thighs (between the hip and knee)
* Front of the thighs
* Calves/front of shin

You should always be careful never to place the foam roller directly on a joint. For example, never apply the roller to your knees or neck. Instead, only place the roller on the solid spaces of your body that have muscle or tissue bulk. When used properly, the foam roller will release trigger points, draw fluid to stiff tissues, and thereby enhance mobility around your joints, which can have positive effects such as improving the range of motion in your hips.

Foam rolling addresses additional body systems:
* Nervous System: Calms your nervous system, which controls tense muscles and tissues.
* Circulatory System: Improves circulation to your extremities, thus warming up the body for activity.
* Connective Tissue: Most abundant substance in the body. Foam rolling is the most effective way to keep this tissue (which is found in cartilage, blood, and organs) healthy.

As previously discussed, the fascia system is an interweaving system of connective tissue wrapping around every portion of the body. Hence, when this support structure is tight or dehydrated (which happens when we age—imagine a dry leaf shriveling up), our joints get tight, muscles don't contract as efficiently, and we generally just don't move well.

When our fascia system becomes tighter and less mobile, our body awareness can decrease. Body awareness is simply sensing how your body interacts within the space around it (car driving by, stepping off a curb) and reacting appropriately. We foam roll because it re-hydrates, gets rid of muscle knots, and creates a greater sense of body awareness.

Physical Benefits from Exercise

Improving Flow of Oxygen, Blood, and Nutrients
By incorporating exercise into a daily routine, anyone can improve their heart rate, which ultimately helps the flow of oxygen, blood, and nutrients to the brain and aids in overall function throughout the body. Being actively involved in exercise over an extended period of time, and on a regular basis, strengthens cartilage in the joints, protects against muscle weakness, and encourages cartilage to self-repair.

Increasing Flexibility and Releasing Tight Muscles
The types of flexibility exercises included in any exercise program should involve a foam roller, isometrics that contract and relax the muscles, and balance training for fall prevention. The Programs (see Chapter 7) in this book combine static and active stretching at the right times, along with the proper warm-up before exercising, to establish a safe and effective routine.

Pain Reduction
Exercise enhances mood by stimulating the release of endorphins. This acts as a natural pain medication, and explains why people generally feel better after 30-45 minutes of physical activity. This can be useful for alleviating chronic joint pain as long as exercises do not cause too much stress on the joints.

CHAPTER FIVE

Rules of the Road: Exercise Precautions

In the following chapter, you will find many great exercises that are ideal for guarding joint health, including exercises that improve balance, strength, and movement-based exercises. The exercises and Programs found in Chapters 6 and 7 are specially designed to be safe and effective, even for those with joint pain.

Patients following the programs in Chapter 7 should not hesitate to cater the program to their own specific needs and abilities by panning through and finding the exercises they really enjoy. These are the exercises you will be more likely to perform with increased regularity and consistency, which are two key factors for achieving a healthier body and healthy joints.

Through performing these exercises, you will be participating in something called *motor learning*. It is important to keep in mind that there will be a learning curve for new physical and mental exercises, which may cause some frustration as you become accustomed to the movements and activities.

The first few weeks of the Program are called the *cognitive (verbal) stage,* during which you will be mentally figuring out what to do. This should last three to four weeks.

During the second learning stage, named the *associative stage,* you should be able to perform the action, but possibly with errors. This should last two to three weeks.

Lastly, the *automatic stage* is when you are able to perform the exercises without error (or, with "great form") and can repeat sets and reps week after week.

Basic Exercise Guidelines

Below are some guideline from the American College of Sports Medicine and the American Heart Association, geared towards healthy populations.

- Build your activity levels slowly and progressively over time. Utilizing the guidance of a fitness professional should be considered.
- Strengthening and stretching muscles can take stress off joints with arthritis pain.
- Break up the amount of time that you workout. Instead of performing 30 minutes of continuous exercise, utilize shorter 10-15 minute segments of swimming, biking, and strength development. Consistency and quality of technique in movements are paramount, quantity can be increased. Work up to fóur to six days per week of moving your body with 45 minutes to1 hour of continuous activity as your goal.
- Fall prevention has become a very important aspect of fitness programming. Exercises that utilize balance, coordination, and multi-tasking (for example, catching a ball while standing on one leg) are becoming more common. Creating confidence in one's movement capabilities leads to greater independence and improved quality of life on a daily basis.
- The body learns through movement, not isolation. Multi-joint exercises such as squatting, dead lifts, pulling, rotational patterns, and extensions (such as prone extension lifts on page 62) teach muscles to work together, ultimately increasing stability of the joints in a more effective way. For example, the muscles in the front and back of the leg (quad/hamstring, respectively) are both working when standing on one leg, hence creating greater coordination between the lower body muscles.

Balance Your Exercises

Dr. Michael J. Hewitt, research director for exercise science at the Canyon Ranch Health Resort in Tucson, Arizona explains that, because skeletal muscles can only contract and are arranged in pairs, exercise programs should have a balance of pulling and pushing movements. He goes on, "One muscle of the pair pulls to bend the joint (flexion), and its antagonist (opposing muscle) pushes to straighten the joint (extension)...Thus a strengthening program must be balanced by pairing every pulling movement with a pushing action (Brody, *New York Times,* 2008)." The exercises in this book provide you with this necessary balance of pulling and pushing, which will help make your workouts more effective.

Exercise Essentials Checklist

Exercise Preparation

- **Exercise Location:** Is your environment safe, clean, and free of debris?
- **Proper Footwear:** Are you wearing proper athletic footwear?
- **Comfortable Athletic Wear:** Do you have clothes that allow freedom of movement?
- **Hydration:** Be sure to drink six glasses of fluid over the course of your day.

Exercise Equipment

- **Rolled-up towel:** Can be used for resistance training, balancing on the floor, etc.
- **Mirror:** Provides visual feedback on cueing and technique
- **Dumbbells:** 5-10 pound range is generally appropriate
- **Therabands:** Light-colored bands offer less resistance and dark-colored bands offer more resistance
- **Physio-ball:** Inflate the ball to the point where you can press your thumb on the surface without it sinking in
- **Tennis ball or racquet ball:** For hand and foot therapy

Playing it Safe: Important Safety Precautions

Body Positioning: Brace your core, achieve proper alignment, feel the placement of your feet, and always move first from your core before moving your limbs.

Keep a Health Journal: In this journal, you can record how you're feeling on any given day and what activities you did during that time. You should also record what kinds of exercises you did on each day and how you felt during and after your exercise session. Keeping track of this information will help you better understand your own health, which is a crucial step on the road to recovery.

Rate of Perceived Exertion (RPE): You can use the chart below to gauge how hard you are working during your session. The corresponding numerical values may also be helpful for you to record in your Health Journal, if you choose to keep one.

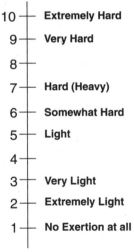

10	Extremely Hard
9	Very Hard
8	
7	Hard (Heavy)
6	Somewhat Hard
5	Light
4	
3	Very Light
2	Extremely Light
1	No Exertion at all

Talk Test: This is another useful way of determining how hard you are working. As you are exercising, gauge how easily you are able to converse and use the guidelines below to figure out the intensity of your exertion.

If you can carry on a normal conversation while exercising, you are likely working *aerobically,* which means your body is using oxygen as its primary energy source. If you can work aerobically for up to 30-45 minutes, your body will also be using fat as an energy source, which is an excellent foundation for building your exercise program.

Anaerobic work, characterized on the following page as medium intensity, should be introduced eight weeks into your exercise program. Examples include hill walking and bike sprints. When performing anaerobic exercise, you may notice your leg muscles starting to feel a bit tight, your chest will expand, you will begin to sweat, and your heart rate will reach about 40-50 beats above your resting heart rate (see page 36 for more details on determining your heart rate).

- **Low Intensity:** Complete sentences, breathing rate normal
- **Medium Intensity:** Broken sentences, breathing rate slightly labored
- **High Intensity:** Cannot converse, breathing rate labored

Be sure to see your healthcare provider regularly for check-ups.

Determining Your Heart Rate

To determine your heart rate, place the tips of your index, second and third fingers on your wrist, below the base of your thumb. You can also place the tips of your index and second fingers on your neck, along either side of your windpipe. During exercise, it is recommended that you find your pulse on your wrist, rather than on your neck.

While pressing lightly with your fingers, you should be able to feel your pulse. If you don't feel your pulse, move your fingers around slightly until you do.

Watch the second hand of a clock or watch and count the number of beats you feel in ten seconds. Using that number, you can calculate your heart rate with the formula below:

(Beats in ten seconds) x 6 = (Heart Rate)

Adults over 18 years of age typically have a resting heart rate of 60-100 beats per minute. To better understand your own heart rate, you should check your pulse before, and immediately after, you exercise. This will give you a better idea of what your body normally does at rest, and to what level your heart should be working during an exercise session.

Calculating Target Heart Rate

Your target heart rate is the level of exertion you should aim for when exercising in order to gain the most benefits from your workout. Your target heart rate is also a useful range for how your body is responding to your workout.

Target heart rate is 60-80% of your maximum heart rate, depending on what level of exertion you wish to work at.

Different Training Zones

Below is a list of the different levels of exertion and the corresponding percentage you would use to reach your target heart rate:

Recovery Zone - 60% to 70%
Active recovery training should fall into this zone (ideally at the lower end). It's also useful for very early pre-season and closed season cross training when the body needs to recover and replenish.

Aerobic Zone - 70% to 80%
Exercising in this zone will help to develop your aerobic system and, in particular, your ability to transport and utilize oxygen. Continuous or rhythmic endurance training, like running and hiking, should fall under this heart rate zone.

Anaerobic Zone – 80% to 90%
Training in this zone will help to improve your body's ability to deal with lactic acid. It may also help to increase your lactate threshold.

To determine your target heart rate, you can use the formulas below to calculate your maximum heart rate, and to then find your target heart rate.

220 – age = maximum heart rate
Maximum heart rate x training % = target heart rate

For example, if a 50 year old woman wishes to train at 70% of her maximum heart rate, she would use the below calculations:

220 – 50 = 170
170 x 70% = 119

She would thus aim to reach a heart rate of 119 during her exercise in order to work at her target heart rate.

You can also use the Karvonen Formula, which is based on both maximum heart rate and resting heart rate. Visit *www.sport-fitnessadvisor.com/heart-rate-reserve.html* for more information.

Important Assessments

Medical Tests

Medical tests include blood panels, neurological/reflexive tests, updated family history, stress test, etc. These are tests that your medical provider can provide based upon your clinical assessment of health and risk profile. Maintain an open dialogue with your medical practitioner, particularly if you have a history of heart problems.

Fitness Tests (Functional and Physical Assessments)

- **Functional Assessment:** The Functional Assessment will provide you with a direct measurement of how you can improve in your activities of daily living. This includes walking stairs, getting in and out of chairs, etc. Refer to Chapter 7, page 94 for the Functional Assessment.
- **Physical Assessment:** The Physical Assessment will provide you with a direct measurement of the improvements you can make in gaining strength as a result of following the exercises in this book. Refer to Chapter 7, page 94 for the Physical Assessment.
- **Waist Size:** To determine your waist-to-height ratio, simply divide your waist size by your height (in inches). A waist-to-height ratio under 50% is generally considered healthy.
- **Stamina:** The average person should be able to walk up a flight of stairs or walk once around an outdoor track without becoming out of breath.
  12-Minute Walking Test: Find a measured distance, such as a track, and see how much distance you can cover in 12 minutes. Make sure you challenge yourself, while still being able to carry on intermittent conversation with a partner (see the Talk Test on page 34). Referring to the Rate of Perceived Exertion (RPE) scale on page 34, you should aim to work at around 5-6 during the first two or three times of repeating this test. Thereafter, challenge yourself to reach a 7-8 on the RPE scale. This test is also known as the Cooper Test. You can complete this on a treadmill, too.
  Quarter Mile Timed Test: Find a measured 400-meter or quarter-mile track. See how long it takes you to cover the specified distance. Aim to work at a 6-7 on the Rate of Perceived Exertion (RPE) scale.
- **Strength:** As you perform the Strength Circuits (see page 100), make note of any improvements you have made. For instance, are you able to perform more reps, or have you continued from beginner to intermediate exercises?

- **Flexibility:** Because levels of flexibility can differ greatly from one individual to the next, it is impossible to provide an average measurement of flexibility. Instead, you should aim to determine what improvements you are making in your Physical Assessment (see page 94) from week to week. This will help you gauge whether you are improving your flexibility based on your body's abilities.

- **Re-Assessment:** Perform the Functional and Physical Assessments again and compare your new results with your original results to determine how much you have improved in your overall strength and function.

Quick Tip: Understanding Your Pain

When you have discomfort somewhere, take a look at the areas above and below the area of discomfort. For example, if your knee has been aching for years, do you notice restricted movement in your hips and ankles? If your lower back is chronically sore, do you have poor posture at your middle back (lower shoulder blade area)? Be proactive about looking above and below the area of discomfort to make sure the joints are doing what they are inherently designed to do, namely to stabilize or move through larger ranges of motion.

CHAPTER SIX

The Exercises

Overhead Squat

Feel it Here Hips, Back, Shoulders

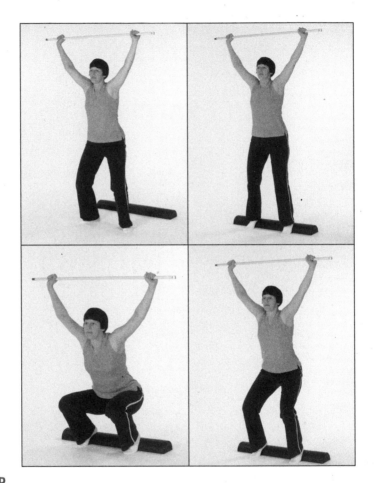

SET-UP

Position yourself with feet hip-width apart. Point your toes to 11 and 1 o'clock positions respectively, as this will allow your hips, knees, and ankles to move together properly during the squatting movement. Place the dowel (broomstick) on the crown of your head so your elbows are at a 90-degree angle, then press the stick above your head. Place a half roller under your heels if you feel your body pitching forward. Drop your hips as low as possible.

Images should be read clockwise.

Getting Up from a Chair

Feel it Here Core

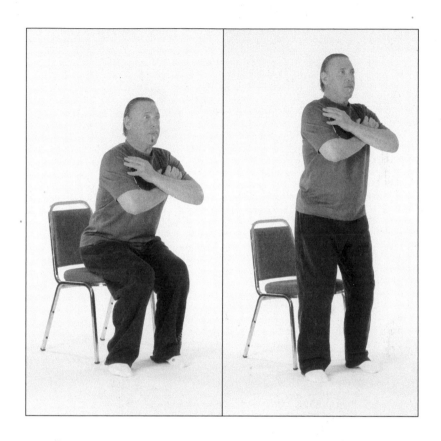

SET-UP

Position yourself on the edge of a chair. Hips should be parallel to, or slightly above, knee level. Brace your core and press your feet into the ground.

Standing with Eyes Closed
Feel it Here Full Body

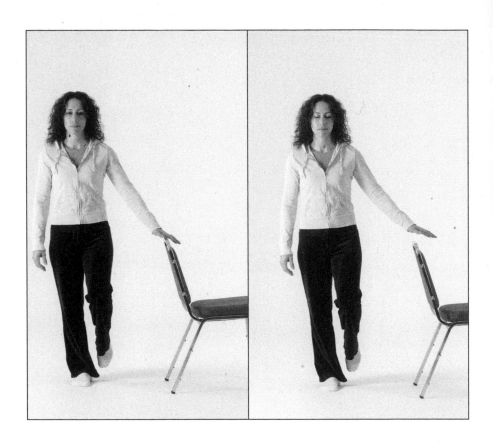

SET-UP

Stand with your feet hip-width apart. You should stand near a wall, chair, or partner for safety. For the two-legged test, rest you hands at your side and close your eyes. With both feet on the ground feel a natural sway similar to a tree in the wind. For the one-legged test, close your eyes once your foot is off the ground. With one foot on the ground the sway will increase dramatically with your body wanting to make very quick readjustments to stabilize.

Heel to Toe Walking

Feel it Here Core, Sides of Legs, Back

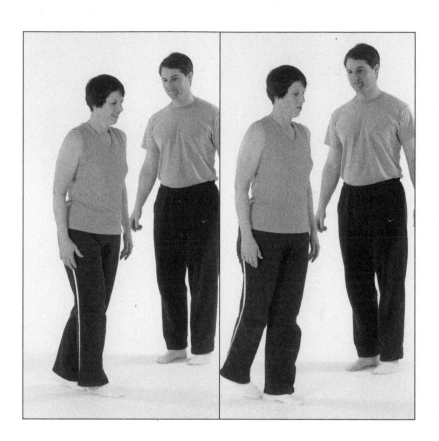

SET-UP

Find a wall or fixed surface prior to beginning this exercise in case you become off balance. Begin with your arms out to the side for added stability. Pick a spot in front of you for focus and begin the movement by placing one foot in front of the other. Experience your upper body attempting to stabilize itself more than when you are in a normal walking position. A dramatic change in stability will occur with one foot in front of, or behind, the other. Take your time and concentrate on the placement of each foot. Repeat backwards toe-to-heel.

Chair Sit

Feel it Here Legs

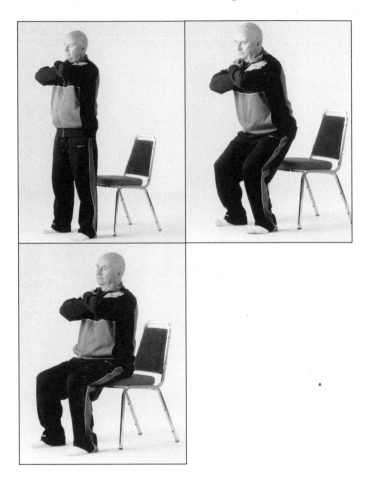

SET-UP

Using the chair as a teaching tool, lower the hips down towards the seat using legs and hips. Hold this position, relax into the chair, repeat. Work on increasing the time held for each rep. A wall can be used if the isometric squat is too much. Position your body against a wall. Walk your hips down the wall by walking your feet out in front of your body. Keep your hips, knees, and toes in line. Maintaining head, shoulder, and tailbone contact with the wall, hold the squatting position as if sitting in a chair. You should not feel pain in your knees. If you do, walk the feet out farther. Breathe into your lower body.

Forward Plank

Feel it Here Stomach, Legs, Shoulders

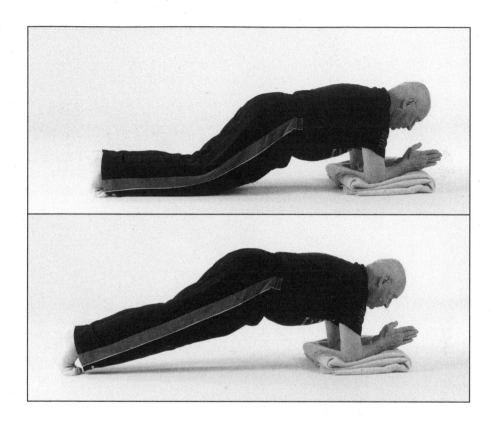

SET-UP
Position your body in the same position as a push-up, but with your hands positioned together in front of your face. To help cue the pulling of the navel to the spine, place a rolled-up towel on your lower back as a bio-feedback tool. Make sure you are breathing through the entire movement. Pull your navel to the lower spine but do not flatten your lower back out. Instead, cue the lower ribs to become 'heavy'.

45

Lateral Plank

Feel it Here Shoulders, Ribs, Obliques, Hip

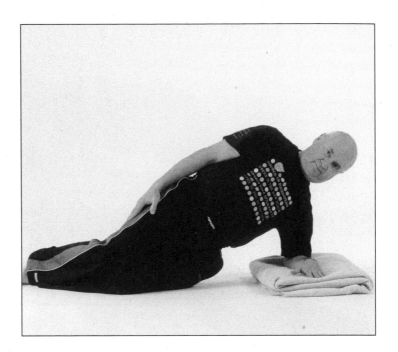

SET-UP

Position your body on one side, on your elbow and hip. Contract the side of your stomach and elevate your hip into alignment with the shoulders and knees.

Lifting Technique

Feel it Here Legs, Stomach, Spine, Shoulders, Arms

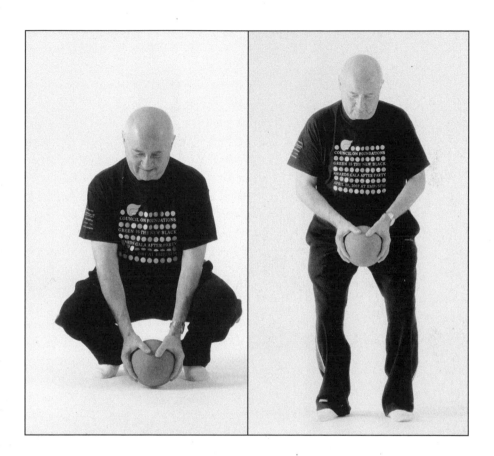

SET-UP

Point your toes to the 11 and 1 o'clock positions. Bend at the hips, knees, and ankles. Keep the object close to your body during the entire motion. Prior to beginning the upward (lifting) movement, brace your stomach and press your feet into the ground, then stand up straight. If you are unable to keep your heels down, it is especially important that you brace your stomach throughout this movement.

47

Rotating Technique

Feel it Here Hips, Middle Back

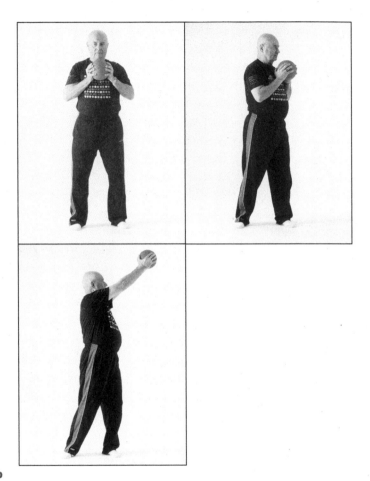

SET-UP
Set up with the same mechanics as for the lifting exercise (see page 47). Keep the object as close as you can until your hips and spine reach their end points. Be careful not to twist through your lower back.

Squatting Technique

Feel it Here Legs, Back

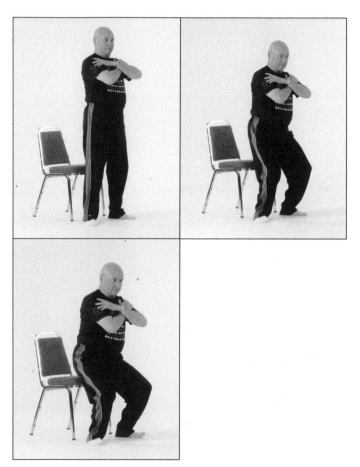

SET-UP

Cross your arms in front of your body. Hands should be resting on the front of your shoulders with elbows relaxed. Brace your stomach. Your toes should be positioned at 11 and 1 o'clock positions to allow proper movement about the hips. Look at a spot on the floor a bit in front of you, but not so much as to be entirely erect. Think about "wrinkling" your groin when squatting. This will force your hips back.

Hip Hinging

Feel it Here Lower Spine, Hamstrings

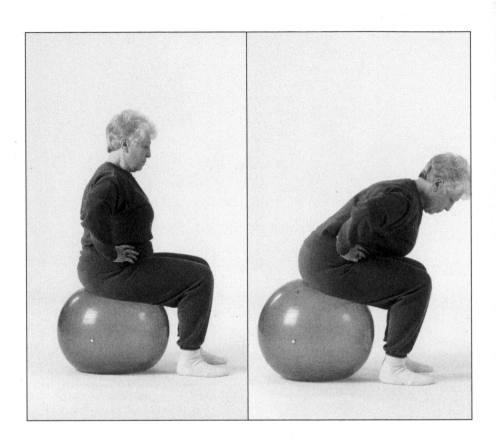

SET-UP
Start the movement from your hips, letting the other parts follow. Feel your upper body positioned over the upper thighs as you "hinge" forward. Brace your stomach, then begin the upward movement, returning to an upright position.

Spinal Whip

Feel it Here Middle Back

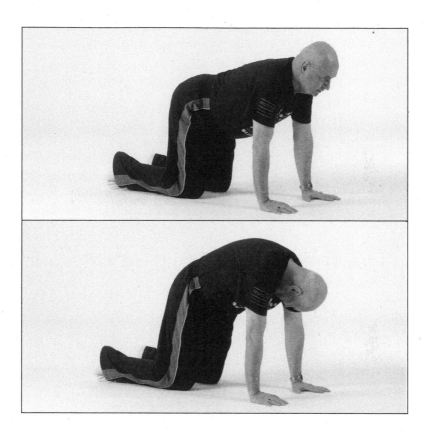

SET-UP

Begin on all fours or standing with your hands on your knees. Rotate from the shoulder blades as they move to the outside of the upper body. Emphasize moving from the middle back through the sternum.

Note: Pay special attention to noticing the difference between your lower, middle, and upper back.

Shoulder Circles

Feel it Here Spine

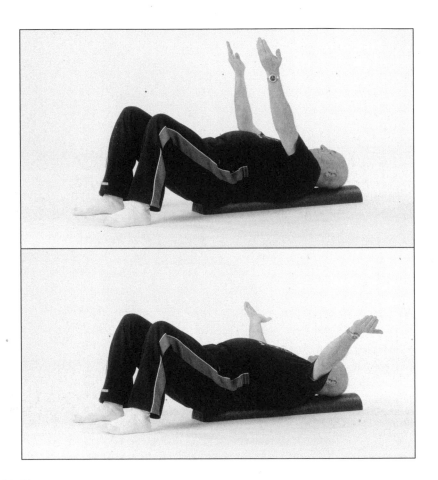

SET-UP

Lay down on the roller with your spine resting in the long position. If you need increased balance during the movement use a half roller or rolled-up towel. Feel pressure on your spine. Only your head, middle back, and pelvis should be resting in contact with the roller. Initiate smooth circles with your arms as if you have a dinner tray in each hand.

Note: This should be attempted using a half roller first and then using a full roller.

Cranial Release

Feel it Here Neck

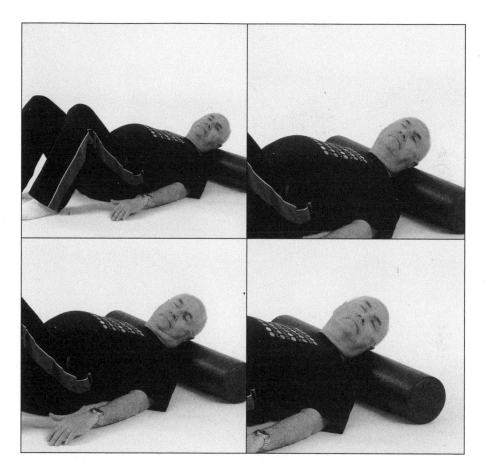

SET-UP

Lay on your back. Position the back of your head, right where it meets the base of your neck, on the roller. You should be in a comfortable position; draw your feet into your hips if needed. Your hands should be relaxed near the sides of your hips. If you need to stabilize the roller, place your hands on the sides of the roller. Rotate your head to the right and left. When rotating your head to the right and left, feel the small space that sits on either side of your head. Keep pressure on the roller by slightly extending your neck, emphasizing proper alignment. *Check out www.meltmethod.com*

Images should be read clockwise.

Sacral Release

Feel it Here · Pelvis

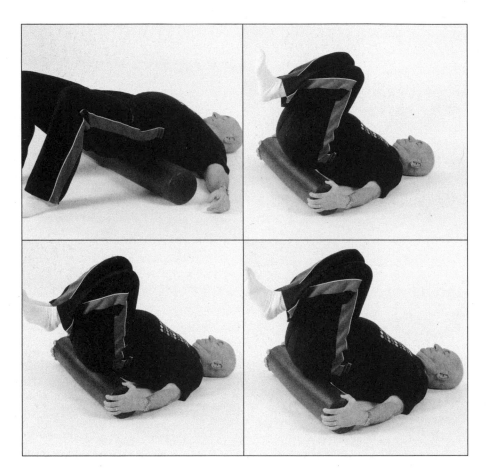

SET-UP

Position your body in a comfortable bridging position on your spine. Elevate your hips and slide the roller on your sacrum. Keeping your ribs heavy, engage your core and pull one knee at a time up to a position over your hips. Addressing one side of your pelvis at a time, let your knees drift over until you feel a 'barrier' or place of irritability. Once found, gently make circles with your knees both ways, then switch to the other side.

Check out www.meltmethod.com

Images should be read clockwise.

MELT Ball Series

Feel it Here Small Joints

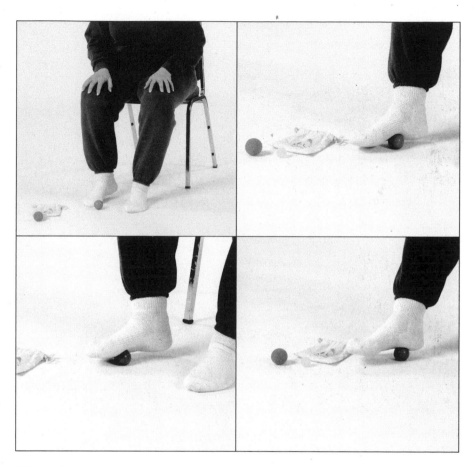

SET-UP

Apply balls to joint and soft surfaces allowing the joints/tissues to decompress and open. Compression is one of our body's enemies as we age. Similar patterns of position point pressing can be applied to the hands. Do not let the balls sink into the soft tissue spaces between the joints—nerves sit there.

Images should be read clockwise.

Ankle Pumps

Feel it Here Front of Shins, Calves

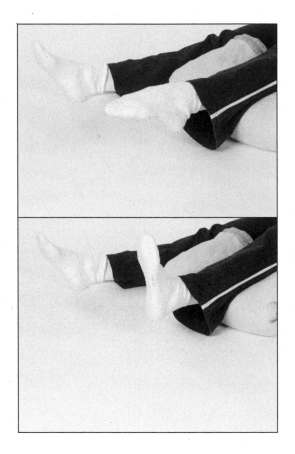

SET-UP

Gently point and flex the foot, reaching out through the front of the big toe.
Pull the toes back by pushing through the heel.

Foam Roller Scissor Stretch

Feel it Here   Core, Lower Back

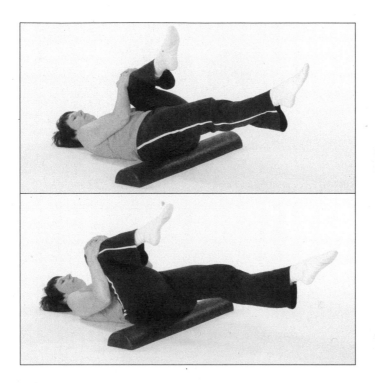

SET-UP

Lay on your back with your knees bent and feet close to your hips. Press your feet into the floor, then elevate your hips. Slide a foam roller (or very thick towel) beneath your tailbone/sacrum. Keeping your ribs heavy, pull one knee to your chest and hold. Extend the leg next, keeping ribs heavy and engaging the core. The sacrum is the flattish bone that positions itself directly below the lower back. Place the palm of your hand on the sacrum; it should fit nicely. The roller sits between the lower back and sacrum. *Check out www.meltmethod.com*

Roll and Hold

Feel it Here Upper and Lower Spine.

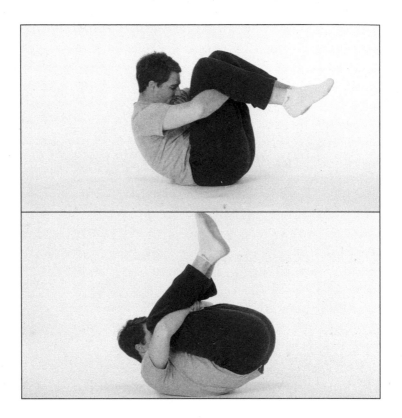

SET-UP
Tuck the knees into your chest and rock back and forth.

Ribcage Opener

Feel it Here Groin, Back, Shoulders

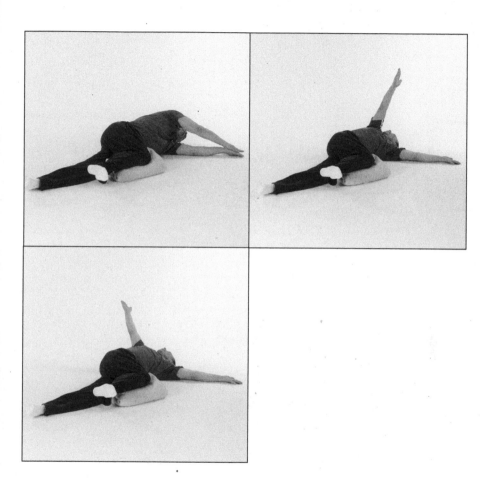

SET-UP

Lay on the ground and position a rolled-up towel or foam roller under your knee. Start with your hands together. Press your knees into the object, then initiate rotation with your hand. Follow the rotation down the arm until you feel it through your ribcage.

Thoracic Flex on Roller

Feel it Here Middle Spine, Abdominals

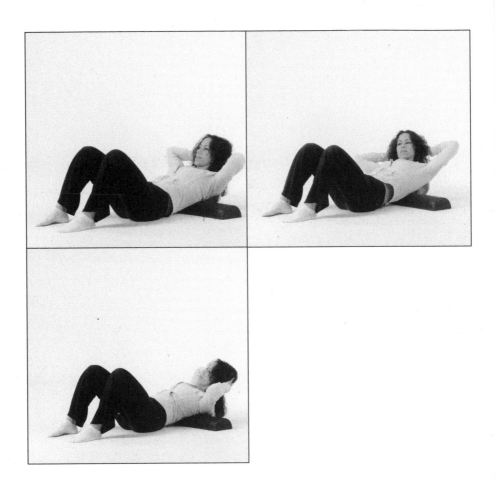

SET-UP

You can use a full roller, half roller, or thick, rolled-up towel. Position the roller immediately below your shoulder blades. Your elbows should be pointed to the sides. Feel the foam roller pressing against your middle spine. Keep your ribs heavy into the ground so the core muscles are active and working through the entire motion. Your front abs will be working the entire time but the latter muscles, namely the obliques, are the actual movers.

Note: This should be attempted using a half roller first and then using a full roller.

60

Physio-Ball Roll

Feel it Here Stomach, Ribs, Chest, Shoulders

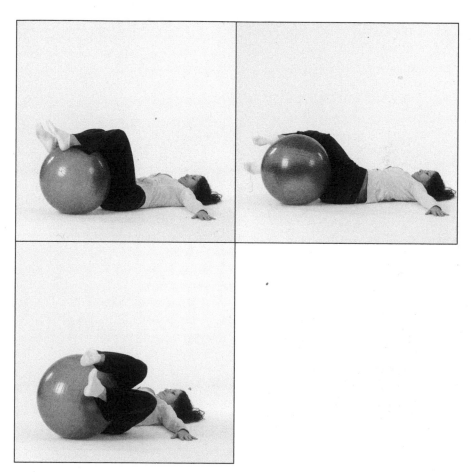

SET-UP

Cup your legs over a physio-ball at an angle slightly greater than 90 degrees, or a square angle at the knees and hips. Position your arms out to the side with palms down to aid in stability during lower body movement. On the way toward the floor, breathe in and gently press the back of your legs into the ball thereby slowing the legs down. On the way back to your starting position, breathe out and press your hand into the floor to activate the stomach and shoulders. This stabilizes your spine prior to moving the ball.

Prone Extension Lifts

Feel it Here Middle and Lower Back, Hips

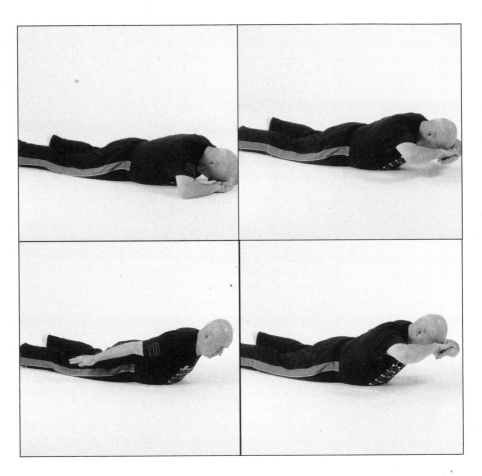

SET-UP

Gently press the front of your lower body into the ground. Initiate the lifting movement from your head, then shoulders, middle back, and lower back. Hold, then release slowly.

Images should be read clockwise.

Heel to Toe Rocks

Feel it Here Full Body

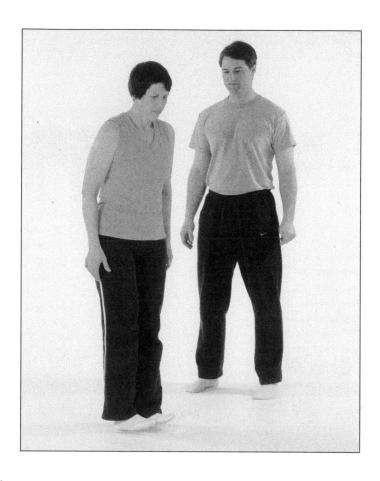

SET-UP

Partner rocks back and forth from the toes to heels as you provide support
if needed.

Physio-Ball Walk-Up

Feel it Here Legs, Hips, Core

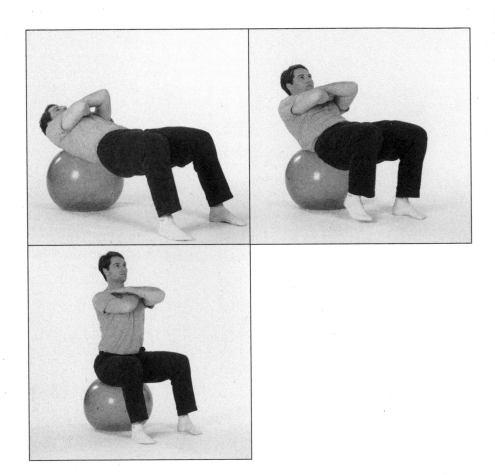

SET-UP

Position your hips on top of the physio-ball. Brace your core. Walk up the ball using your full foot. Keeping the feet wider adds stability if you feel off-balance during the up or down phases.

Lateral Ball Roll

Feel it Here Glutes, Legs, Spine

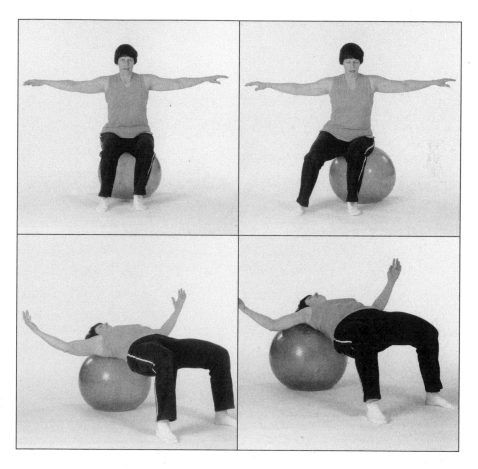

SET-UP

Begin sitting upright on the physio-ball. Keep your feet in front of your hips and "walk" to the left on the ball. Repeat to the right side. The on-back version will be completed in the same manner, but your beginning position will be on your back.

Clock Series: Single Foot Touches

Feel it Here Legs, Hips

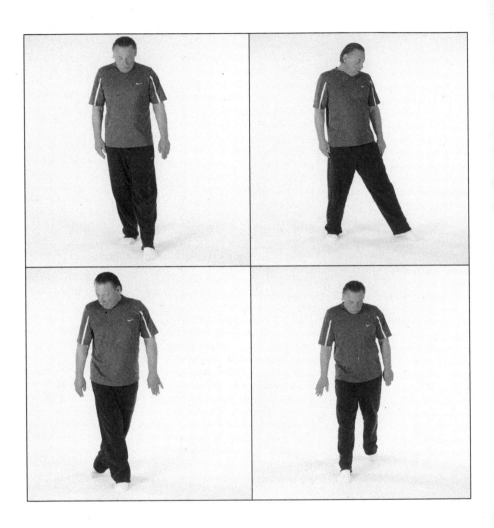

SET-UP

Imagine you are standing in the center of a clock face. Touch two to three numbers around the clock. As you become more comfortable, touch more numbers, then switch feet.

Images should be read clockwise.

66

Clock Lunge

Feel it Here   Hips, Legs

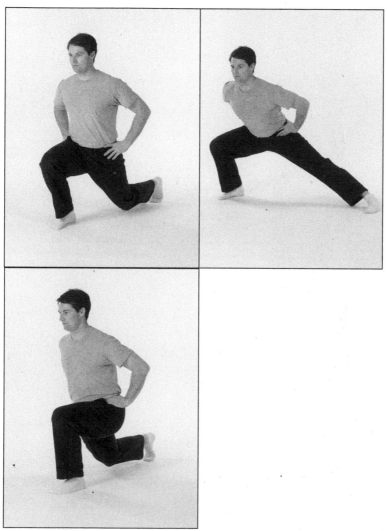

SET-UP

Imagine you are standing in the middle of a clock face. Lunge to various positions on the clock face. Lunging needs to be executed with proper
movement at the hip and knee. Sit the hips down and back into each number on the clock face.

Balancing on Half Roller

Feel it Here Hips, Quads, Calves

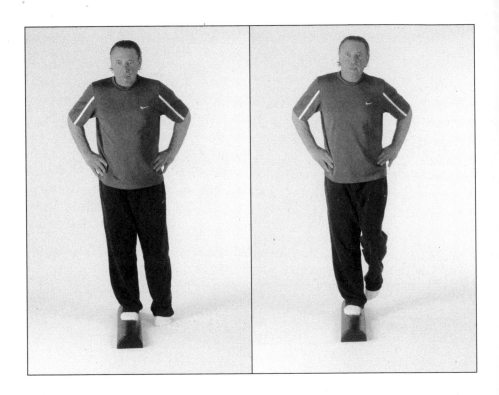

SET-UP

Step onto the roller, keeping both feet on the ground. Gently pick one foot up off the ground. Expect your opposite ankle to feel unstable. Keep your core braced.

Inch Worm Walk-Up

Feel it Here Shoulders, Core, Legs

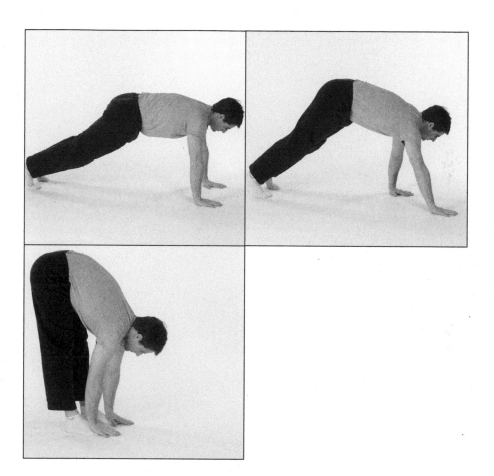

SET-UP

Beginning in a pike position, walk your hands forward until you reach the starting position for a push-up. Brace your stomach, then walk your hands back toward the feet. Do not allow your back to sag once the push-up position is reached. Keeping your hands moving together during this movement is important.

Double Leg Bridge

Feel it Here Back of Legs, Hips, Back

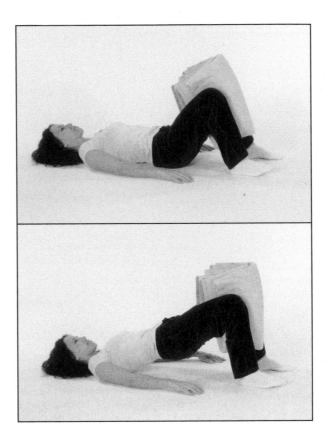

SET-UP

Starting on your back, press the feet into the ground to feel the leg muscles contract. Brace your core, then lift the hips to form an alignment between the knees, hips, and shoulders.

Single Leg Bridge

Feel it Here Hip, Lower Back

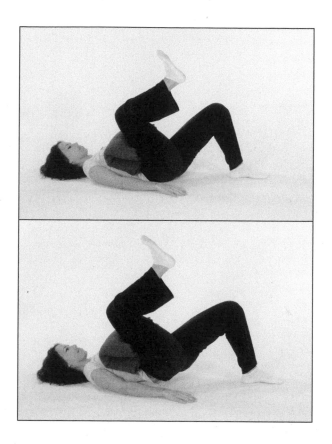

SET-UP

Starting on your back, press your foot into the ground to feel your leg muscles contract, particularly in the hip and hamstring. Brace your core, then lift your hips to align your knee, hip, and shoulder.

71

Band Rows

Feel it Here Middle Back, Arms

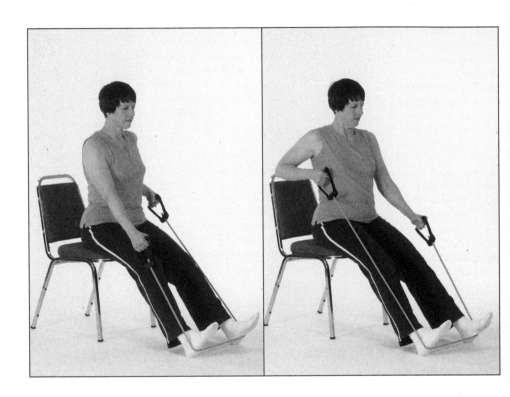

SET-UP

Execute the movement by drawing one elbow back while 'punching' the opposite arm forward. The objective is to learn rotation and build strength in the traditionally weak core and shoulder girdle. This is important for posture, during walking and sitting. If you feel discomfort in your neck, concentrate on relaxing the shoulder blades back and down.

Band Pulls with One Knee Up

Feel it Here Core, Arms, Chest, Legs

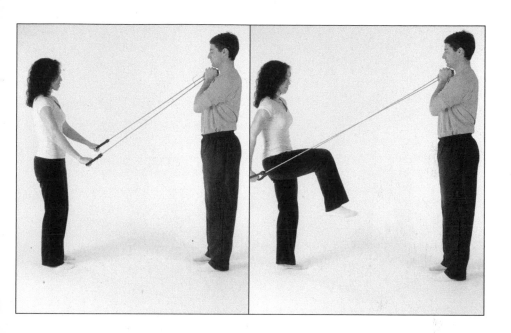

SET-UP

In a standing position, pull your knee upward towards your chest while pulling the arms to the sides of your body. Keep your ribs heavy and core contracted during each pressing repetition. Breathe out during each pressing rep and breathe in upon returning to the starting position.

Alphabet Series: W's

Feel it Here Middle Back

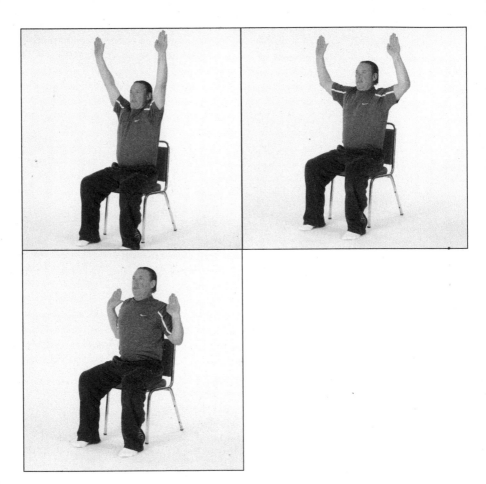

SET-UP
Sit upright on a chair or sturdy surface. Squeeze your shoulder blades back and down. Draw both elbows down and back into the middle spine. Hold, then release.

Alphabet Series: Y's

Feel it Here Middle and Lower Back

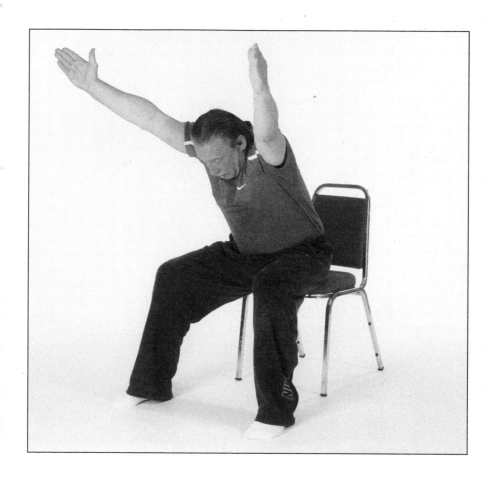

SET-UP
Sit upright on a chair or sturdy surface. Squeeze your shoulder blades back and down. Draw both arms up, and straight out in front of your body at a 45 degree angle.

Alphabet Series: T's

Feel it Here Middle Back, Behind Shoulders

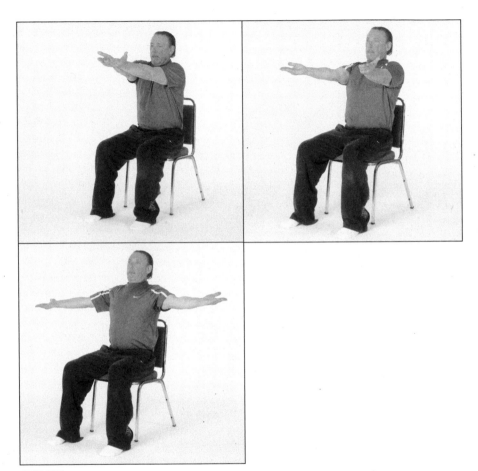

SET-UP

Sit upright on a chair or sturdy surface. Squeeze your shoulder blades back and down. Draw both arms out from the mid-line of the body with palms up.

Stability Hold in Push-Up

Feel it Here Core, Shoulders, Legs

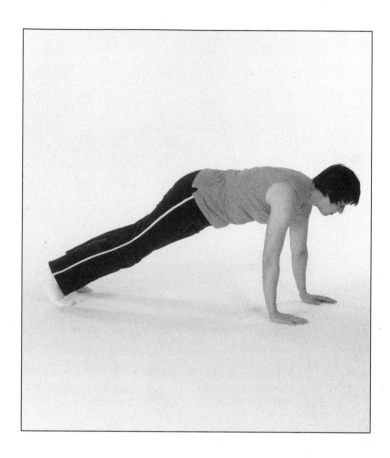

SET-UP

Assume a push-up position. Brace your core, be strong through your spine, and remain balanced on your hands and feet.

Physio-Ball Rotational Twists

Feel it Here Spine, Back

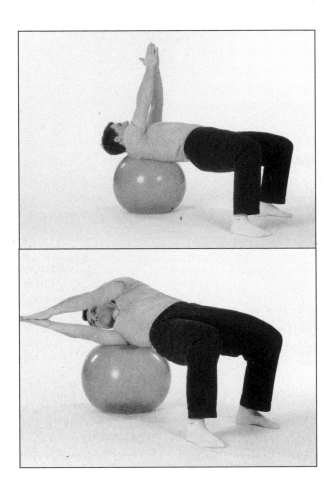

SET-UP

Sit on the highest point of the physio-ball. Keeping your feet steady, walk down until your shoulders and head are resting comfortably on the ball. You will be positioned in a bridge position with emphasis placed on the hips, feet, and back muscles for stability. Keep the hips up by imagining you're squeezing a piece of paper between your glutes, which flattens out the hips. Don't let your hips drop! Press your hands together and initiate the twisting movement from your shoulders and core until your shoulders are stacked. Stacking the shoulders will indicate you've reached your end point.

Standard Lunge with Bicep Curl

Feel it Here Stomach, Obliques

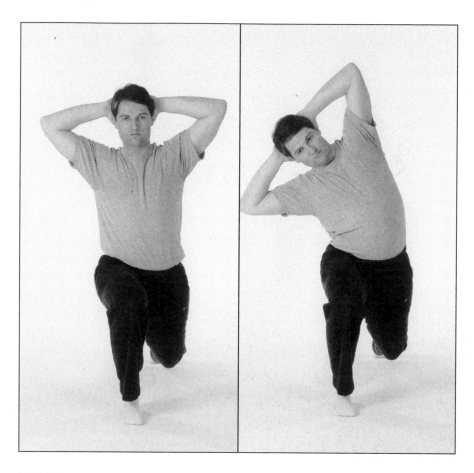

SET-UP

Lunging is nothing more than an exaggerated step. For an advanced lunge (shown, right), make sure your hips are stable and then flex your trunk to the same side as the front leg. Begin to initiate the bicep curl once your lunging motion is completed.

Deadlift

Feel it Here Hips, Legs, Back

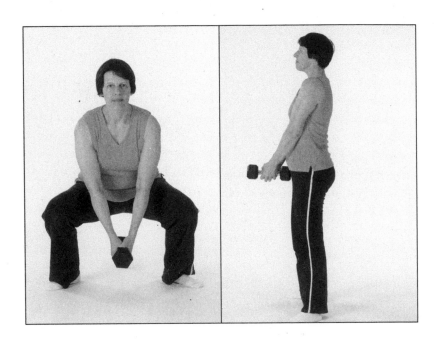

SET-UP

Squat with a dumbbell between your legs and perform the deadlift, slowly lifting the dumbbell up as you straighten your legs.

Band Presses with Two Arms

Feel it Here Chest, Shoulders, Arms

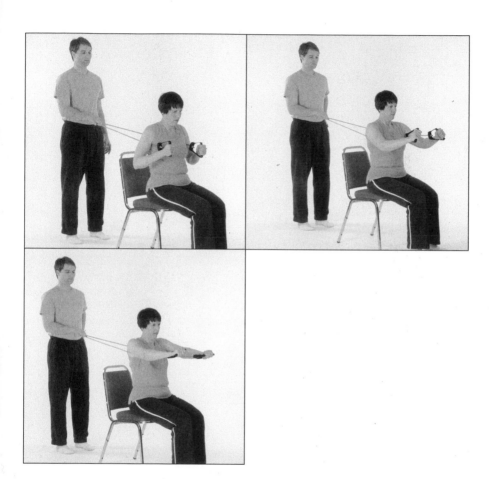

SET-UP

Position your body in a standing position in a normal stance or a split stance. Press your hands out in front until your elbows are fully extended. Keep the ribs heavy and core contracted during each pressing repetition. Breathe out during each extension and breathe in upon returning to the starting position. This exercise can also be done while sitting (shown above) in an upright position on either a chair, ball or a bench.

Chopping Movements

Feel it Here Core, Hips

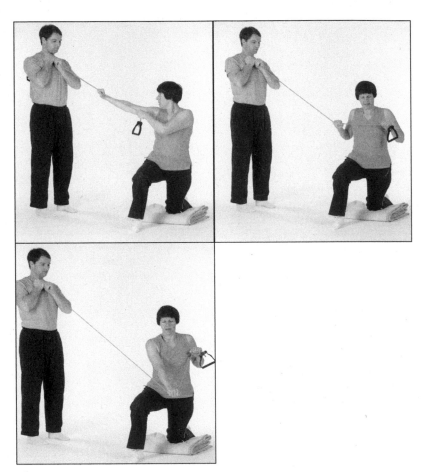

SET-UP

Chop across your body over a trailing, kneeling leg. Your front knee is on
the ground on a towel or other comfortable item. Pull the band into your
body, then push it down and out with the trail hand. Keep your spine neutral
by concentrating on bracing your stomach and stabilizing the hips. Think
about moving around a stable pillar in your spine.
Exercise provided by St. John's, AAHFRP, FMS

Lifting Movements

Feel it Here Core, Hips

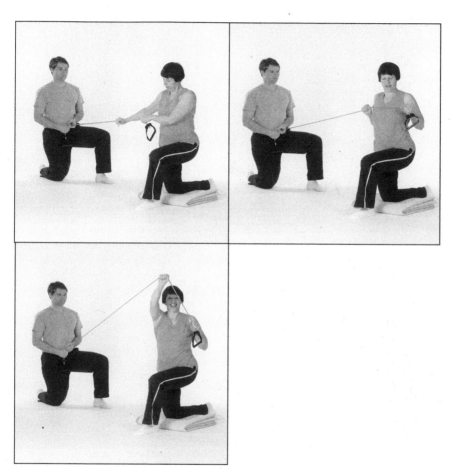

SET-UP

You will be lifting across your body over a trailing knee on the ground. The front knee should be aligned with your hip. Pull the band into your body, then push it up and out with the trailing hand. Keep your spine neutral by concentrating on bracing your stomach and stabilizing the hips. Think about moving around a stable pillar in your spine.

Exercise provided by St. John's, AAHFRP, FMS

83

Push-Up

Feel it Here Stomach, Chest, Arms, Legs

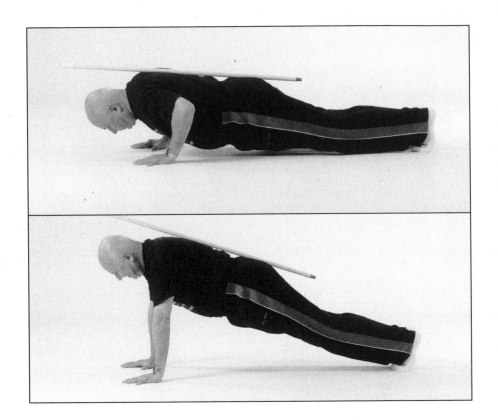

SET-UP

Position yourself on your stomach. Your hands should be parallel to your shoulders. Place a dowel stick along the spine so contact is made with your head and sacrum. Begin the movement by bracing your stomach. Push your toes and hands into the floor, then attempt to press your body away from the floor until your elbows are straight. You should feel your shoulder blades come together as you return to your starting position. To make this exercise increasingly difficult, pick up one foot at a time while keeping your knees straight, but not locked.

Lateral Lunge with Shoulder Press

Feel it Here Hips, Knees, Ankles

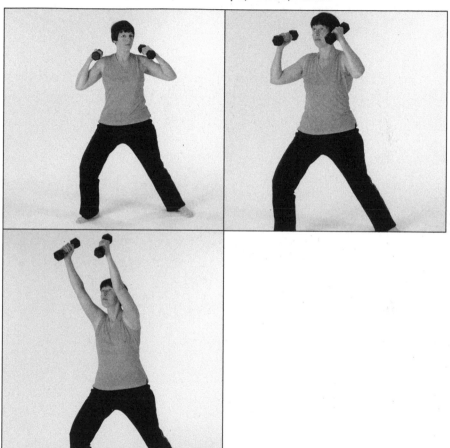

SET-UP

Lunge to the side, sitting back into the exercise. Upon reaching the ending position of the lunge, perform the shoulder press by pressing up and slightly across your body. Upon returning to the starting position, reset the dumbbells to the original starting position. Be sure to keep your back straight and your shoulders squared, and make sure to remain facing the same direction while lunging.

Chest Stretch Open Arms

Feel it Here Chest, Shoulders

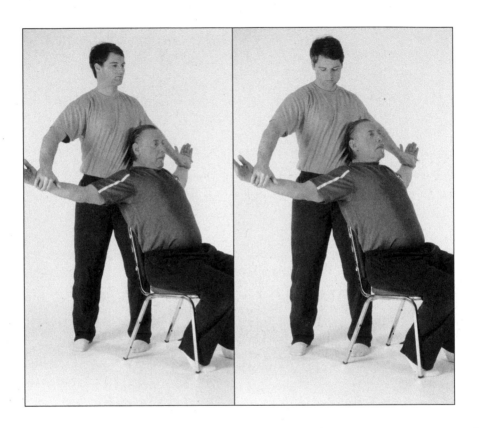

SET-UP

Stand behind your partner with your hands gently placed upon his or her upper arms. Keep your body positioned along your partner's spine to stabilize and assist in creating a greater stretch through the front of your partner's body.

Partner Stability Pushes

Feel it Here Core, Spine

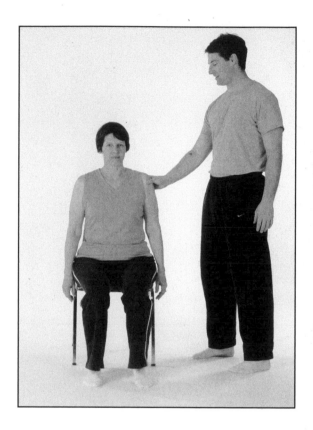

SET-UP

Your partner will start in a seated position. Instruct him or her to breathe during the entire exercise. Proceed to gently push at the shoulders, middle back, and front of the body.

Lateral Shoulder Raises

Feel it Here Shoulders

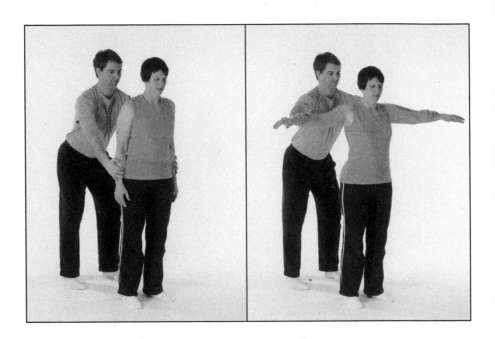

SET-UP

Your partner begins in a standing position. Instruct him or her to make soft fists while pushing into your resistance. Resistance is applied on the upward motion only.

Back to Back Butterfly Stretch

Feel it Here Groin, Hips

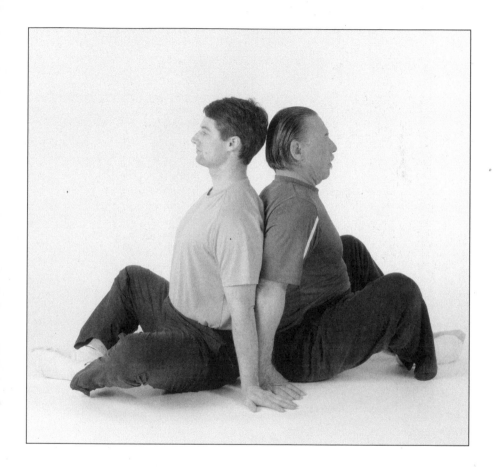

SET-UP

Sit back-to-back with your partner in the butterfly position, with your legs
out to the side to stretch your inner thighs and hips.

Assisted Apley Stretch

Feel it Here Arms, Shoulders, Chest

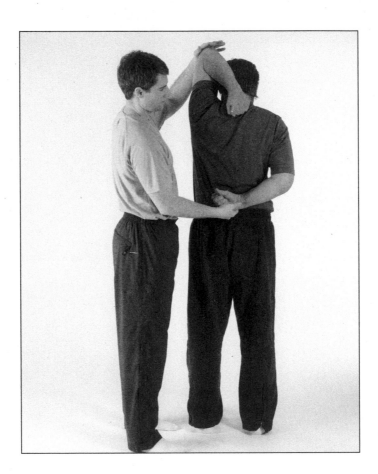

SET-UP

Instruct your partner to reach his or her arms over and under their shoulder blades, as shown above. Assist the elbows coming together while instructing your partner not to arch the middle back.

CHAPTER SEVEN

Exercise Programs and Progressions

Programs

Introductory
AM
- Start the Self-Treatment and Massage progression (see page 96)
- Start the Posture Basics progression (see page 95)

PM
- Weekly: Finish the initial Functional Assessment (see page 94)

Beginner Healthy Joints Program
AM
- Start the Movement: Balance progression (see page 98)
- Start the Beginner Strength progression (see page 100)
- Start the Beginner Movement: Mobility progression (see page 97)

PM
- Practice the Movement: Balance progression (see page 98)

Intermediate
AM
- Start the Intermediate Strength progression (see page 101) or the Stability progression (see page 99)
- Practice Self-Treatment and Massage progression (see page 96)
- Practice the Movement: Balance progression (see page 98)

PM
- Practice the Movement: Balance progression (see page 98)
- Practice your favorite Movement: Mobility progression (see page 97)

Advanced

AM

- Practice the Movement: Balance progression (see page 98)
- Re-test your Physical Fitness Assessment (see page 94)
- Practice the Intermediate Strength progression (see page 101)

PM

- Practice the Movement: Balance progression (see page 98)

Supplemental Program

- Start the Techniques progression (see page 95)
- Start the Partner Workouts progression (see page 102)

Progressions

Rest refers to the time taken between each set of exercises.

RPE refers to Rate of Perceived Exertion. See page 34 for details.

Assessments

INITIAL EVALUATION DATE (WEEK 1):

MID-POINT EVALUATION DATE (WEEK 4):

SUMMARY EVALUATION DATE (WEEK 9):

FUNCTIONAL ASSESSMENT	COMPLETE (Yes/No)	DISCOMFORT (Yes/No)	NOTE DIFFICULTY
Overhead Squat			
Standing with Eyes Closed (two legs)			
Standing with Eyes Closed (one leg)			
Heel to Toe Walking			
Getting Up from a Chair			

PHYSICAL FITNESS ASSESSMENT	GOAL	INITIAL	MID-POINT	SUMMARY
Chair Sit	1 Minute			
Forward Plank	45 Secs			
Lateral Plank	45 Secs			
12-Minute Walking Test (page 37)				

Techniques

Reps: 10
Sets: 2
RPE: 5/10

Exercise	Page #	Equipment
Lifting Technique	47	weighted object
Rotating Technique	48	weighted object
Squatting Technique	49	chair

Posture Basics

Reps: 15
Sets: 1
RPE: 3/10

Exercise	Page #	Equipment
Hip Hinging	50	physio-ball
Spinal Whip	51	
Shoulder Circles	52	foam roller or rolled towel

Self-Treatment and Massage

Reps: 15
Sets: 1
RPE: 2/10

Exercise	Page #	Equipment
Cranial Release	53	foam roller or rolled towel
Sacral Release	54	foam roller or rolled towel
MELT Ball Series	55	small ball

Movement: Mobility
Beginner Segment
Reps: 12
Sets: 1-2
RPE: 4/10

Exercise	Page #	Equipment
Ankle Pumps	56	foam roller or rolled towel
Foam Roller Scissor Stretch	57	foam roller or rolled towel
Prone Extension Lifts	62	

Intermediate Segment
Reps: 12
Sets: 1
RPE: 4/10

Exercise	Page #	Equipment
Roll and Hold	58	
Ribcage Opener	59	foam roller or rolled towel
Thoracic Flex on Roller	60	foam roller or rolled towel
Physio-Ball Roll	61	physio-ball

Movement: Balance

Reps/Seconds: 10
Sets: 2
RPE: 5/10

Exercise	Page #	Equipment
Clock Lunge	67	
Physio-Ball Walk-Up	64	physio-ball
Lateral Ball Roll	65	physio-ball
Balancing on Half Roller	68	half roller or rolled towel
Clock Series: Single Foot Touches	66	
Heel to Toe Rocks	63	

Stability

Reps: 10
Sets: 2
RPE: 6/10

Exercise	Page #	Equipment
Inch Worm Walk-Up	69	
Double Leg Bridge	70	rolled towel

Strength

Beginner Segment: Lower Body
Reps: 12
Sets: 2
RPE: 6/10

Exercise	Page #	Equipment
Single Leg Bridge	71	rolled towel
Band Rows	72	theraband, chair
Alphabet Series	74-76	chair
Lifting Movement	83	theraband, towel

Beginner Segment: Upper Body
Reps: 12
Sets: 2
RPE: 6/10

Exercise	Page #	Equipment
Band Rows	72	theraband, chair
Band Pulls with One Knee Up	73	theraband
Alphabet Series	74-76	chair
Stability Hold in Push-Up	77	dumbell

Intermediate Segment: Lower Body/Core
Reps: 10
Sets: 2-3
RPE: 7/10

Exercise	Page #	Equipment
Physio-Ball Rotational Twists	78	physio-ball
Standard Lunge with Bicep Curl	79	
Band Pulls with One Knee Up	73	theraband
Deadlift	80	dumbbell

Intermediate Segment: Upper Body/Core
Reps: 12
Sets: 3
RPE: 6-7/10

Exercise	Page #	Equipment
Push-Up	84	dowel stick
Lateral Lunge with Shoulder Press	85	dumbbells
Chopping Movement	82	theraband, towel
Band Presses with Two Arms	81	theraband, chair

Partner Workouts

Reps: 12
Sets: 1-2
RPE: 5/10

Exercise	Page #	Equipment
Chest Stretch Open Arms	86	chair
Partner Stability Pushes	87	chair
Lateral Shoulder Raises	88	
Back to Back Butterfly Stretch	89	
Assisted Apley Stretch	90	

GLOSSARY

Ankle Joint
A synovial hinge joint that occurs where the foot and the leg meet. This joint is composed of the tibia, fibula, and talus.

Arthritis
Term used for a group of more than 100 medical conditions that affect the musculoskeletal system, specifically where two or more bones meet to form joints. Arthritis-related joint problems include pain, stiffness, inflammation, and damage to joint cartilage and surrounding structures.

Biomechanics
The study of biological systems (specifically their function and structure), based on principles of traditional engineering sciences.

Blood Pressure
The pressure blood exerts on the arteries. Produced mainly by heart muscle contractions, blood pressure is measured by two numbers. Systolic pressure is higher and taken after the heart contracts. Diastolic pressure is lower and taken before the heart contracts.

Brain and Spinal Cord
The portion of the nervous system containing the brain and the spinal cord that is responsible for coordinating the body's activity.

Cervical Spine
Consisting of seven vertebrae with eight pairs of cervical nerves, the cervical spine begins at the base of the skull, making up the first section of the spine. The individual cervical vertebrae are abbreviated as C1, C2, C3, C4, C5, C6, and C7.

Compression Stress
A decrease in volume or compacting of space. For example, pressing your hands together.

Compound Joint Movement
Any movement that simultaneously utilizes several muscles or muscle groups.

Connective Tissue
A material made up of fibers forming a framework and support structure for body tissues and organs. Connective tissue surrounds many organs. Cartilage and bone are specialized forms of connective tissue. It has recently been shown that certain forms of connective tissue have contractile-like properties.

Core
An umbrella term used to define the neuro-muscular system that is located between the shoulders and knees. Technically, "core" is a limiting term because the body learns through movement, not isolation. Hence, using the entire body during exercises activates your core.

Diagonal Pattern
Spiral pattern of movement.

Diaphragm
Primary respiratory muscle that wraps over the liver and stomach. The heart touches the diaphragm upon each beating contraction.

Extension Pattern
Increases the angle between the bones at the joint.

Flexion Pattern
Decreases the angle between the bones at a joint.

Frontal Plane
A vertical plane running from side to side that divides the body (or any of its parts) into anterior and posterior portions.

Hip Joint
The joint located between the femur and acetabulum. This joint functions to support the weight of the body and maintain balance.

Intervertebral Discs
Tough, dense bundles of cartilage cushions that serve as the spine's shock absorbing system. The intervertebral discs give protection to the vertebrae, brain, and other structures such as the nerves. While individual disc movement is very limited, together the discs allow for some extension and flexion.

Isolated Joint Movement
Any movement that utilizes one muscle or muscle group at a time.

Joint-by-Joint Theory
A theory developed by Gray Cook and Michael Boyle, which states that each joint in the body fulfills a specific function, alternating between mobility and stability as you move further up the body.

Knee Joint
A synovial hinge joint which joins the thigh and leg. This joint consists of four bones—the femur, tibia, fibula, and patella.

Lumbar Spine
The largest segment of the vertebral column, most people have five lumbar vertebrae, although it is not unusual to have six. Making up the lower portion of the back, the lumbar vertebrae are larger than the cervical or thoracic as this spinal region carries most of the body's weight.

Lumbo-Sacral Complex
The area in the body that includes the lower back (lumbar spine) and sacrum (pelvic region). Common movements such as walking, running, squatting, and lunging involve this area of the body.

Mobility
This term relates to both joints and global movement capacity. Each joint is meant to have proper mobility through its range of motion, whereby humans must have effective mobility to walk, run, and perform activities of daily living. Mobility is a major problem as we age.

Myofascial System
"Myo" means muscle and "fascia", as defined by Dr. Ida P. Rolf, is "An elastic fabric, subjected to pull of any sort, transmits the strain in many directions over a wide area. If the displacement exceeds the elastic limits, an aberrant pattern remains." Together, "myo" and "fascia" come to mean a whole-body functioning system of movement.

Orthostatic Hypotension
A decrease of blood pressure that may occur when standing or exercising, characterized by acute dizziness, blurred vision, and/or weakness.

Peripheral Nervous System

The peripheral nervous system extends outside of the central nervous system. Its main function is to connect the body (limbs and organs) to the central nervous system, thereby executing necessary movement functions.

Proprioception

Often referred to as the "sixth sense," the nervous system developed proprioception to keep track of, and control, the different parts of the body.

Posture

How you position your body upright against gravity when standing, sitting or lying down. To have good posture requires teaching your body how to stand, sit and lie in ways that minimal strain is put on the muscles and ligaments used while moving or doing weight-bearing activities (Cleveland Clinic).

Resting Heart Rate

This is a person's heart rate at rest. The best time to find your resting heart rate is in the morning after a good night's sleep, and before you get out of bed. According to the American Heart Association, the heart beats about 60 to 80 times per minute while at rest.

Rotation Pattern

Masses articulating atop one another through the transverse plane. For example, think of placing your arms on a table top. Slide your arms back and forth—that's the transverse plane.

Sacrum

The large, triangular-shaped bone that consists of the five fused vertebrae below the lumbar region. The spinal canal extends into the sacrum and the sacral nerves exit the canal through an opening in the bone. There is also a wedge-shaped intervertebral disc between the base of the last lumbar vertebra and the sacrum, which is called the lumbosacral disc.

Sacroiliac Joints

Occurs where the sacrum is joined with the ilium, or top portion of the pelvis, on both sides of the back. These joints bear the weight of the twists and turns of the body's trunk.

Sagittal Plane

A vertical plane running from front to back that divides the body (or any of its parts) into right and left sides.

Shearing Stress
A sliding type of stress. For example, surfaces rubbing together creates friction.

Shoulder Joint
Occurs where the humerus meets the scapula. The shoulder is comprised of three joints—the glenohumeral, acromioclavicular, and sternoclavicular joints.

Spinal Cord
A large, thin, almost circular bunch of nerve tissue that carries messages or sensations from the brain to the rest of the body and vice versa. At each level of the spine, except the top cervical vertebrae, the spinal cord branches into paired nerve roots that leave through spaces (neural foramina) located between each vertebra.

Spine
The spinal column is one of the most vital parts of the human body, supporting the trunk and making all of our movements possible. Protection, communication, and sensation are a few of the spine's functions. The spinal cord is located inside the vertebral (spinal) column.

Stability
The quality, state, or degree of being stable.

Stamina
Resistance to fatigue, illness, and hardship; endurance.

Tensile Stress
An increase in the length of a structure. For example, pulling your finger away from your hand.

Thoracic Spine
Located in the chest area and having 12 vertebrae, the thoracic spine attaches to the ribs, protecting vital organs.

Torquing Stress
Rotating type of stress. For example, turning a door knob.

Transverse Plane
A horizontal plane that divides the body (or any of its parts) into upper and lower parts.

Vertebrae
The average person is born with about 33 individual bones (the vertebrae) that interact and connect with each other through flexible joints, or facets. By the time a person becomes an adult, most have only 24 vertebrae because some vertebrae at the bottom end of the spine fuse together during normal development.

Vertebral Foramen
Open space that allows nerves, amongst other structures, to leave their origin.

ABOUT THE AUTHORS

William Smith, MS, NSCA, CSCS, MEPD, completed his B.S. in exercise science at Western Michigan University followed by a master's degree in education and a post-graduate program at Rutgers University. In 1993, Will began coaching triathletes and working with athletes and post-rehab clientele. He was a Division I Collegiate Strength Coach and has been competing in triathlons and marathons since 1998, recently finishing the Steelhead Half Ironman in Michigan in 5 hours and 22 minutes. Will founded Will Power and Fitness Associates and currently consults for fitness, healthcare, and wellness centers in New York and New Jersey. The Director of the Professional Development Institute, Will has also co-authored a book on triathalon training (*Tri-Power*, 2007).

Jo Brielyn is a freelance writer and author. She is a contributing writer for Hatherleigh Press and has published works in several print and online publications. Jo also owns and maintains the Creative Kids Ideas (www. creativekidsideas.com) and Good for Your Health (www.good-for-your-health.com) websites. For more information about Jo's upcoming projects or to contact her, visit www.JoBrielyn.com. Jo resides in Central Florida with her husband and two daughters.

Mary Jane Myslinski, EdD, EdM, MA, PT received a Baccalaureate degree in Physical Therapy from Boston University in 1977 and a Master of Arts in Cardiopulmonary Rehab from New York University in 1982. She did further graduate work at Columbia University receiving an EdM in 1989 and an EdD in Applied Physiology in 1995. Dr. Myslinski's academic and research interests are in the relationship between aerobic/anaerobic exercise and physiological function in patients with disabilities or chronic disease. Her clinical practice focuses on patients with orthopedic and neurologic problems.

Also in the *Exercises for* Series...

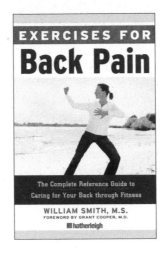

Exercises for Back Pain
ISBN 978-1-57826-304-2

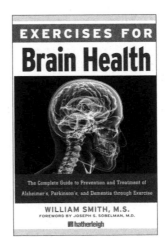

Exercises for Brain Health
ISBN 978-1-57826-316-5

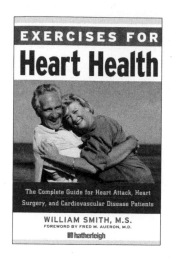

Exercises for Heart Health
ISBN 978-1-57826-303-5

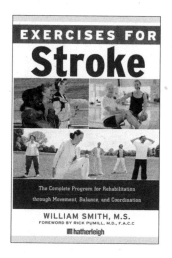

Exercises for Stroke
ISBN 978-1-57826-317-2

MY FITNESS NOTES

MY FITNESS NOTES

MY FITNESS NOTES

_____
_____
_____
_____
_____
_____
_____
_____
_____
_____
_____
_____
_____
_____
_____
_____
_____
_____
_____
_____
_____
_____
_____

MY FITNESS NOTES

MY FITNESS GOALS

MY FITNESS GOALS

_____

_____

_____

_____

_____

_____

_____

_____

_____

_____

_____

_____

_____

_____

_____

_____

_____

_____

_____

_____

_____

MY FITNESS GOALS

_____
_____
_____
_____
_____
_____
_____
_____
_____
_____
_____
_____
_____
_____
_____
_____
_____
_____
_____
_____
_____
_____
_____

MY FITNESS GOALS

_____

_____

_____

_____

_____

_____

_____

_____

_____

_____

_____

_____

_____

_____

_____

_____

_____

_____

_____

_____

_____

_____

_____

MY FITNESS GOALS

_____

_____

_____

_____

_____

_____

_____

_____

_____

_____

_____

_____

_____

_____

_____

_____

_____

_____

_____

_____

_____

_____

_____

_____

_____

_____

MY FITNESS GOALS

_____

_____

_____

_____

_____

_____

_____

_____

_____

_____

_____

_____

_____

_____

_____

_____

_____

_____

_____

_____

_____

_____

_____

_____

IN EARLY JUNE 1964,

the Benevolent Home for Necessitous Girls
burns to the ground, and its vulnerable residents
are thrust out into the world. The orphans, who
know no other home, find their lives changed
in an instant. Arrangements are made for the
youngest residents, but the seven oldest girls
are sent on their way with little more than a clue
or two to their pasts and the hope of learning
about the families they have never known.
On their own for the first time in their lives,
they are about to experience the world in ways
they never imagined...

MY LIFE BEFORE ME

Norah McClintock

ORCA BOOK PUBLISHERS

Library and Archives Canada Cataloguing in Publication

McClintock, Norah, author
My life before me / Norah McClintock.
(Secrets)

Issued in print, electronic and audio disc formats.
ISBN 978-1-4598-0662-7 (pbk.).—ISBN 978-1-4598-0663-4 (pdf).—
ISBN 978-1-4598-0664-1 (epub).—ISBN 978-1-4598-1092-1 (audio disc)

I. Title. II. Series: Secrets (Victoria, B.C.)
PS8575.C62M85 2015   jc813'.54   c2015-901738-6
         c2015-901739-4   c2015-901740-8

First published in the United States, 2015
Library of Congress Control Number: 2015935517

Summary: In this YA novel, would-be reporter Cady investigates racism and
family secrets in a small Indiana town.

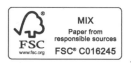

*Orca Book Publishers is dedicated to preserving the environment and has
printed this book on Forest Stewardship Council® certified paper.*

Orca Book Publishers gratefully acknowledges the support for its publishing
programs provided by the following agencies: the Government of Canada through
the Canada Book Fund and the Canada Council for the Arts, and the Province of British
Columbia through the BC Arts Council and the Book Publishing Tax Credit.

Cover design by Teresa Bubela
Cover images by Dreamstime.com and Shutterstock.com

ORCA BOOK PUBLISHERS
www.orcabook.com

Printed and bound in Canada.

18 17 16 15 • 4 3 2 1